HOW TO LIVE WELL
WITH DIABETES

A Comprehensive Guide to Taking Control
of Your Life with Diabetes

HOW TO LIVE WELL WITH DIABETES

A Comprehensive Guide to Taking Control of Your Life with Diabetes

Dr Val Wilson

A How To book

ROBINSON

ROBINSON

First published in Great Britain in 2019 by Robinson

1 3 5 7 9 10 8 6 4 2

A CIP catalogue record for this book
is available from the British Library.

Important information
This book is not intended as a substitute for medical advice or treatment.
Any person with a condition requiring medical attention should consult a
qualified medical practitioner or suitable therapist.

ISBN: 978-1-47214-405-8

Typeset by Initial Typesetting Services, Edinburgh
Printed and bound in Great Britain by Clays Ltd, Elcograf S.p.A.

Papers used by Robinson are from well-managed forests and other responsible sources.

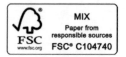

Robinson
An imprint of
Little, Brown Book Group
Carmelite House
50 Victoria Embankment
London EC4Y 0DZ

An Hachette UK Company
www.hachette.co.uk

www.littlebrown.co.uk

How To Books are published by Robinson, an imprint of Little, Brown Book
Group. We welcome proposals from authors who have first-hand experience
of their subjects. Please set out the aims of your book, its target market and its
suggested contents in an email to howto@littlebrown.co.uk.

Contents

About this book

This book has been written to help you understand your diagnosis so you can manage and live well with your diabetes for as long as possible. The knowledge in this book has been acquired over forty years from many sources, for which I'm very grateful. Everything you need to know is covered in each chapter with important words in italics – they also appear in the glossary at the end of the book, accompanied by a more detailed explanation. I have included loads of facts and tips that appear in bold throughout, and there's an extensive index that you will hopefully find useful. I have also frequently used case studies to convey other people's experiences of diabetes-related issues that you might be experiencing, too.

I can honestly say that you never stop learning when you have diabetes and everything there is to learn is not always simple. There's blood glucose – BG – monitoring to consider, and medication, diet and exercise to get to grips with – a complete lifestyle change. *How to Live Well with Diabetes: A Comprehensive Guide to Taking Control of Your Life with Diabetes* gives you answers to making these changes so you can be in control of your diabetes rather than it being in control of you.

Introduction

There has never been a better time in history to be diagnosed with either Type 1 or Type 2 diabetes. I was recently reminded of this while watching a TV advert during a prime-time show for a swipe-technology glucose-testing machine, available to buy over the Internet and now accessible in most counties of the UK on the NHS. Thankfully, we've moved on from the way things used to be. Even forty years ago there wasn't the knowledge that high glucose levels cause other health problems. I'll say it again – we are so lucky to be able to use available knowledge and technology to prevent or delay complications of diabetes in this day and age!

In 1977, when I was aged ten and diagnosed with *Type 1 diabetes*, I had no idea what diabetes was nor what it meant for my future, so I didn't really care about looking after the condition. I did my two injections of *insulin* per day using a glass syringe and stainless-steel needle that had to be sharpened on a pumice stone and sterilised in surgical spirit; and I did a urine test for glucose every morning and evening – that was that. If the urine test turned orange, I knew I was in trouble, but there was no advice about reducing a high blood-sugar – glucose – level. I saw a diabetes specialist once a year who said my condition was incredibly difficult to control, and I was advised that if I did any sport at school, I needed to eat a chocolate bar beforehand. That was the sum total of the diabetes care I received forty years ago.

There is a phrase, 'Laughter is the best medicine'. Well, it is, but I'd rank insulin – the hormone that controls blood glucose levels – or *Metformin*, prescribed to manage *Type 2 diabetes*, right up there, too. 'So, having available treatments is brilliant,' I hear you cry. It certainly is and I, for one, wouldn't be here without them. But there is, unfortunately, a cruel irony; a bittersweet twist: by staying alive longer with available treatments for diabetes, the consequences of long-term, higher-than-normal blood glucose – BG – levels can cause complications.

Believe me, this is not one of those slap-on-the-wrist warnings that you should look after yourself (or else!), without explaining why or how. I know from personal experience that the finger-wagging approach to managing diabetes can send a person running and screaming for cover. This is how it was in the 1970s, when I was often on the receiving end of tellings-off. What I hope to do in this book is explain what diabetes is, and why and how you can manage it to prevent or significantly delay the development of any complications. The ultimate goal for me is to provide you with insight, experience and information so you can lead a happy, healthy life with diabetes.

Chapter 1

So, What *Is* Diabetes?

Diabetes is a change in your body chemistry that causes too much glucose in the blood. This is because of a lack of the hormone insulin, or because insulin can't work properly in the body. There are two kinds of diabetes:

TYPE 1 DIABETES happens when the body attacks its own insulin-producing cells in the *pancreas* so that your body makes little or no insulin at all. This is a permanent situation and the exact cause is unknown, but viral and genetic factors are thought to play a part. In other words, Type 1 diabetes can't be cured.

TYPE 2 DIABETES is a complex condition involving a number of factors, including high blood glucose levels. It is usually triggered by excess body weight and a lack of physical activity. With this condition, there is usually a combined alteration in the amount of insulin produced when blood glucose levels are too high, and a reduced response to insulin in the body cells so that the hormone can't do its job properly.

Although the medical profession may disagree with me, I've always believed that the best person to educate others about diabetes is someone who actually has the condition because 'you don't get it until you get it'. This does, of course, depend on the teacher and their own understanding of the condition: in 1850, for example, a diabetes consultant advised his patients that they needed to eat vast quantities of *sugar* to replace what was being lost in their urine! The irony was he was also diabetic – his own treatment killed him and most of his patients.

If you're wondering what makes me such an expert – you already know that I'm someone with long-term diabetes – I also have a doctorate qualification in diabetes health education. Initially, I studied this area with the intention of helping myself rather than other people, but I soon found my knowledge was useful for others, too.

Case study: Dave

Dave had recently been diagnosed with Type 2 diabetes. Dave was tired, thirsty, taking frequent trips to the toilet to empty his bladder, and began experiencing blurred vision and numbness in his feet and lower legs. He'd ignored these symptoms for several months, putting them down to just getting older. During a routine visit to the dentist, Dave was advised to go and see his GP because high glucose levels had led to thrush – a yeast infection – in his mouth. A few weeks later, Dave was finally diagnosed with Type 2 diabetes and began taking Metformin tablets to lower his BG levels. He felt better almost immediately, but because he felt better, Dave thought his diabetes had gone away. One day, Dave's wife told me, 'He's so much better now, but he feels ill if he eats a few doughnuts.' Sadly, no one had told Dave about avoiding sweet foods unless he had the symptoms of low BG such as dizziness, sweating, shaking and confusion. I explained that taking Metformin does not mean Type 2 diabetes goes away, or that if he took a tablet Dave could eat sweet foods as he had done before he had diabetes. Dave said he hadn't known what or who to ask as his doctor and nurse were busy, with little time to make things clear.

Needing to visit the bathroom more often and having a raging thirst are major symptoms of diabetes, although this can be much less obvious in Type 2 diabetes and can last for years before diagnosis, compared with the dramatic thirst and urination seen prior to diagnosis in Type 1. In the seventeenth century, diabetes was described as 'the pissing evil' – remembering that there was no treatment at the time. This sums up perfectly the relentless flow of urine caused by too much glucose in the system. The thirst and need to urinate happens because the body is trying to flush out all the excess glucose that it can't use without the help of insulin (or glucose-lowering tablets) to convert it to energy.

As I've mentioned, there are two main types of diabetes that happen for different reasons, but both ultimately lead to increased BG levels if left untreated. Type 1 diabetes is very quick to develop. If BG levels become dangerously high, this may lead to a medical emergency. According to Diabetes UK, Type 2 diabetes may take up to twelve years to develop fully, but because the level of glucose in the blood is higher than normal over a prolonged period of time, complications such as heart disease may occur. Imagine the heart trying to pump thick syrup around the body and you can see why keeping BG levels under control is so important: high BG thickens the blood and makes it sticky. To recap:

TYPE 1 DIABETES happens when the body no longer produces the hormone insulin to control BG levels because the insulin-producing part of the pancreas is attacked by the body's own defence mechanisms – an auto-immune attack. This is a life-long, irreversible condition and used to be called 'child onset diabetes' because it mainly happens in younger people.

TYPE 2 DIABETES is a different form of the condition with its own causes and effects. It is a complex disorder that results in the body not being able to use insulin to bring BG levels under control. This used to be seen most often in people over forty years of age, especially the elderly where the pancreas had begun to wear out. Today, Type 2 diabetes is recognised as a condition related to lifestyle, as it is often seen in people who are overweight and inactive. The body produces more and more insulin to attempt to bring BG levels down, but the fat surrounding body cells means the body can't use this insulin properly. In most cases, lifestyle changes, such as weight loss and regular exercise, can reverse this imbalance. It's a sad fact that because of an inactive lifestyle, Type 2 diabetes in children is now steadily increasing.

> **FACT:** You may think that Type 2 diabetes is not as serious as Type 1. This is not the case. Having Type 2 diabetes increases the risk of developing heart disease, so having good control of BG, blood pressure and *cholesterol* levels is very important.

There are two other forms of diabetes worth mentioning here:

GESTATIONAL DIABETES develops in the mother from the twentieth week of pregnancy because hormonal changes block the normal action of insulin in the mother's body. The effect disappears after the baby has been born. However, more than half of women who have had gestational diabetes will have an increased risk of developing Type 2 diabetes within 15 years of the pregnancy.

DIABETES INSIPIDUS is a rare condition carrying the symptoms of increased thirst and frequent urination, but, when tested, the blood and urine do not contain an abnormal amount of glucose.

Chapter 2

How Many People Have Diabetes?

Don't worry – if you have diabetes, you are not alone and needn't suffer in silence. Around 700 people a day are diagnosed with diabetes – that's the equivalent of one every two minutes. In January 2016, Diabetes UK announced that four million people now have diabetes of one form or another in the UK. Globally, this figure is currently 415 million, although this does not include children with the condition.

Because Type 2 diabetes is usually related to lifestyle and people today can expect to live longer with serious medical conditions that can be managed, this form of diabetes accounts for 90 per cent of cases. The remaining 10 per cent have Type 1 diabetes, but this too is on the increase.

There are an estimated 31,500 children and young people with diabetes in the UK, meaning around two in every thousand children have diabetes – the majority with Type 1. This estimate is based on the number attending diabetes clinics specifically for young people, but the figure could be as high as 42,000 because some 15–19-year-olds attend an adult diabetes clinic. Around 95 per cent of these children and young adults have Type 1 and the remainder have Type 2 diabetes. In the year 2000, the first cases of Type 2 diabetes were diagnosed in overweight female children as young as 7 years old. There are slightly more boys than girls with Type 1, but more girls than boys develop Type 2.

> FACT: GP surgeries now offer annual health checks in which you can take a urine sample to be tested for glucose, even if you haven't had any symptoms of diabetes.

Type 2 diabetes in the UK is usually managed by you and your GP as opposed to a diabetes consultant at a hospital. This is called *Primary Care*. This is to make sure you are looked after by health professionals who can help you keep good control of your BG, blood pressure and cholesterol to reduce the risk of developing any of the complications of diabetes. Getting your diabetes care from a GP and Practice Nurse has the main advantage of allowing you to phone for an appointment whenever you need it rather than just seeing a diabetes consultant every six months or yearly. Your GP surgery also has easy access to your medical notes and history and they know you better than a more impersonal hospital clinic, where you may not see the same health professional each time you have an appointment and will have to repeatedly explain details about your diabetes. Attending several different clinics can be tiresome – medical notes are not shared between hospitals.

How many people don't know they have diabetes?

Because Type 2 diabetes is developing so often in what is known as 'Western society', where people eat a high-*calorie*, high-fat diet and do little or no exercise, the condition has reached epidemic proportions worldwide. The symptoms are mild and can often be ignored for years before diagnosis.

Experts think that one person in every sixteen now has Type 2 diabetes without knowing it. Like Dave, mentioned in the earlier case study, the symptoms may be put down to getting older or being tired because of work or life stresses. The trouble with having high BG levels over many months, or even years, is that this can eventually cause damage to blood vessels and nerves – and there are blood vessels and nerves all over the body, so any part of you can be affected by diabetes. This means it's important to go to your doctor with any symptoms – like an increased thirst or frequent visits to the toilet – to get a diagnosis as soon as possible.

Chapter 3

Living With Diabetes

'The worst thing for me was being told that I'd have diabetes for the rest of my life.'

So, you have diabetes? You may be feeling depressed and angry, thinking 'Why me?' This is a perfectly normal reaction. What is different in your case is that you've made the first positive step towards taking control by buying this book. The way you deal with your diabetes is very personal and it's never too late to start having a better understanding of how it affects you – knowledge is your greatest weapon. This can be the difference between diabetes becoming a condition that rules your life or a condition you are confident you can manage.

Symptoms

You may wonder why I'm mentioning the symptoms of diabetes when you've already been through this bit, had your diagnosis and have begun taking medication. The reason this section is here is because diabetes can do far less damage to the body if it is diagnosed early and you are in a position to be able to help someone else who hasn't yet had their diagnosis, but may have some of the symptoms of diabetes – which may be different from your own.

Case study: Natalie

Paula Brown noticed that her 10-year-old daughter, Natalie, seemed to be drinking more and was very tired all the time. Paula was worried that Natalie had lost a lot of weight rather quickly, although she had actually been eating more, saying she was hungry. After a few weeks Natalie began to wet the bed, even though she was emptying her bladder before she went to sleep. Paula mentioned these symptoms to the family GP, but he reassured her that it was probably only a urine or bladder infection and that Natalie should be given plenty of fluids. After a fortnight, Natalie's symptoms seemed worse and Paula took her to see a different GP in the practice. He did a urine test and told Paula that it contained a high amount of glucose. Natalie was admitted to hospital and diagnosed with Type 1 diabetes. She was started on insulin injections to bring her glucose levels under control. After seeing the hospital diabetes nurse, Natalie began to manage her Type 1 diabetes very successfully at home and at school.

Case study: John

John Taylor was 55, overweight and took little exercise. His job as a security guard required that he would sit and watch CCTV footage for most of the day. He was feeling itchy much of the time and his wife, Maureen, thought he might be having a reaction to their washing powder, so she changed it. Four months passed and John was now feeling he had no energy, despite drinking a bottle of Lucozade – liquid glucose – every day. As time went on, John convinced himself he felt under the weather because of the stresses and strains of his job. John hated visiting his GP as the doctor always commented on his weight, so he forced himself to keep going without seeing anyone. One weekend about a year after John first complained of constant itching, he collapsed while mowing his front lawn. Maureen called an ambulance and, after tests at the hospital, John was told he had Type 2 diabetes. Maureen wished she'd encouraged John to see his doctor about the itching.

As you can see, Natalie and John both had very different symptoms. Type 1 diabetes tends to make itself known within weeks or months, whereas Type 2 diabetes – with more subtle symptoms that are often easy to ignore – can take many years.

What are the main symptoms of diabetes?

Feeling very thirsty and needing to urinate far more frequently than usual are the main symptoms, which occur because your body cannot deal with excess glucose. This is because your body is not producing insulin if you have Type 1 diabetes or because your body can't use insulin properly in Type 2 diabetes. As a result, glucose levels build up in the blood, and the excess then enters the urine. The body produces more urine, so we need to go to the toilet more often. We feel more frequently thirsty and drink more to replace the fluids and flush the glucose out. The only treatment for these symptoms is to replace the insulin by injection, or to take glucose-lowering medication.

Thirst and a need to urinate (especially at night) are not, however, the only symptoms. As well as these, you may have experienced all or only some of the following before diagnosis:

- Dehydration through loss of fluids.
- Tiredness and lethargy.
- Blurred vision.
- General itching and an increase in episodes of *thrush* – a yeast infection.
- Weight loss.

WHY GLUCOSE IS THE ISSUE

Your body uses glucose for energy to power your brain, muscles and the chemical reactions that control ordinary body functions. *Glucose* is a type of sugar that comes from the breakdown of carbohydrates like bread, potatoes and pasta. *Sugar* is a simple carbohydrate that breaks down into glucose in the body. Eating either glucose or sugar – or the carbohydrates that become them as they are processed by the body – increases BG levels.

The pancreas (an organ in the abdomen) releases the hormone insulin into the bloodstream to control the level of glucose. Imagine insulin as the burly doorman that allows glucose to enter into muscle or fat cells. Although there is plenty of glucose waiting to get into the cells, without insulin there is no way of letting the glucose through. The cells become starved, which is why people with Type 1 diabetes often experience rapid weight loss before diagnosis. With Type 2 diabetes where there is obesity, the fat around body cells stops insulin working correctly, so the body produces more and more insulin, but it can't do its job. Whichever type of diabetes you have, your body needs insulin in order for your cells to function and keep you healthy.

FACT: As well as controlling BG levels, insulin supports the formation of fat and muscle; it enables the storage of glucose in the liver as *glycogen* for later use; and it prevents *protein*, needed for cell growth, from being broken down.

When your doctor tells you that you have diabetes, your tests have shown excessive glucose levels in your blood owing to inadequate available insulin. Glucose in the blood is measured in millimoles per litre – mmol/L. I talk about your own BG tests to self-manage diabetes later, but in terms of diagnosis, doctors will use any one of the following results to decide whether or not someone has diabetes:

- A glucose level in a blood plasma sample – the liquid part of blood – of 11 *mmol/L* or higher.
- A BG measurement of 6.1 mmol/L after the person has fasted for ten hours and drunk only water.

- A *glucose tolerance test* showing a plasma glucose level higher than 11 mmol/L two hours after drinking 75g of glucose dissolved in water.

If you have high BG levels but with no symptoms of diabetes, such as increased thirst and a need to urinate more often, you will need a second test to confirm a diagnosis of diabetes.

FACT: Being overweight means insulin can't work properly in the cells of the body. This is called *insulin resistance.*

Diagnosis – Why me?

To answer the question 'Why me?' we have to go into personal matters such as pre-existing medical conditions, genetic factors and lifestyle issues that make a person more likely to develop diabetes. Medical conditions – such as certain cancers – that require the removal of part of the pancreas increase the likelihood of a person developing diabetes, but it's less severe, because the hormone glycogen – which raises BG levels in the body – is also reduced, meaning you can function with less insulin.

Other auto-immune conditions are often diagnosed before or after Type 1 diabetes. These include under- and over-active thyroid conditions; asthma; *coeliac disease* (an intolerance to gluten); and *psoriasis* (a condition affecting the skin).

Genetic factors

Having a parent with Type 1 diabetes increases the odds of also developing diabetes by 3–4 per cent. If you have an identical twin with Type 1, you have a 20 per cent chance of also getting the condition, but this drops to 5 per cent if you have a non-identical twin. If you have a sibling of a different age (that is you are not a twin or other multiple baby), and he or she has the condition, you have a less than 1-per-cent chance of also developing Type 1 diabetes.

In terms of Type 2 diabetes, having an identical twin with the condition means you have a 90-per-cent chance of also developing it. If one of your parents has Type 2, you are 40 per cent more likely to also develop the condition in your lifetime and if both your parents have Type 2, this likelihood rises to 50 per cent.

Racial and ethnic minorities – defined as American Indians and Alaska Americans; Black or African Americans; Hispanics or Latins; and Asian Americans – are more likely to develop diabetes than Whites and some minority groups. Figures show that Type 2 diabetes develops more often in the Asian population, with 16 per cent of Asians in the UK affected.

Existing medical conditions

Medical conditions causing increased levels of other hormones can have a significant effect on the way insulin works, meaning the body has to produce more insulin to make BG levels normal – *glucose intolerance*, and diabetes may develop owing to genetic factors. If you are prescribed anti-inflammatory medicines such as hydrocortisone or Prednisone for conditions such as severe asthma, arthritis, or inflammatory bowel disease, this could increase your chances of developing diabetes.

Certain drugs can also have the side effect of increasing BG levels. These include some blood-pressure medications, especially *Bendrofluozide*, and the water tablets, Thiazide, which raise BG levels and can lead to diabetes if you are genetically susceptible to developing the condition.

Lifestyle

Lifestyle factors such as being overweight and having a high Body Mass Index (BMI), as well as doing little or no exercise, mean you are much more likely to develop Type 2 diabetes than if you maintain a healthy weight and are physically active. We know this because people who live in countries where the population doesn't traditionally eat fast food or junk food, and where people are very active, tend to have a much lower risk of developing Type 2 diabetes.

Asian populations that went from eating fish and vegetables to eating higher fat, higher calorie foods have gone on to have a 60-per-cent increase in the occurrence of Type 2 diabetes. This means that changing your life-style from eating healthy foods and being active to eating convenience foods and junk foods that tend to be high in calories and fat can, over time and in combination with little or no exercise, make you much more likely to develop Type 2 diabetes at some time in your life.

BMI: Your BMI is a measurement that uses your height and weight to work out if you're healthy, although this can be a problem for people with a large amount of muscle – like rugby players, as muscle is heavier than fat. A person with a BMI of 20–24.9 is considered to be of normal weight whereas a BMI of 25–29.9 is classed as overweight. A BMI of 30 and above is considered obese. To calculate your BMI, divide your weight in kilograms by the square of your height in metres. For example, if you are a man who is 1.83 metres tall weighing 90 kilograms, your BMI is 27.

Studies have shown that people with a BMI of 35 and above are 100 times more likely to develop Type 2 diabetes than people with a BMI of 22 or lower. The length of time that a person is obese is also important: the longer they are obese, the more likely they are to develop Type 2 diabetes.

FACT: If you are a woman with a waist measurement of over 89cm owing to excess fat around your middle, or a man whose waist measures over 101cm because of excess fat in this area, you are at an increased risk of developing Type 2 diabetes and heart disease.

EXERCISE: Having a *sedentary lifestyle* – meaning taking little or no exercise – significantly increases your chance of developing Type 2 diabetes, especially in association with obesity. Even if someone is slim, Type 2 can still occur if they take little or no exercise. Studies show that a Type 2 diagnosis happens far more often in people who do not exercise than in those who are fairly active.

OBESITY: A key factor indicating an increased risk of developing Type 2 diabetes is the excess body fat that sits around the waistline, making the person appear apple-shaped rather than pear-shaped. Insulin cannot work properly when there is a lot of fat present around the body cells and excess fat in the mid-section of the body has the greatest effect on the working ability of insulin to reduce BG levels.

The good news is that fat around the waist – known as *visceral fat* – is much easier to lose when you diet than fat elsewhere in the body. This is because when you reduce your calorie intake and become more physically active, your body first uses up the fat stored in this area for energy. Make sure you consult your doctor if you're planning to start dieting and before beginning a new exercise regime.

Case study: Joan

Joan Ralph was 44 and worked in an office. She had recently put on weight after eating takeaway meals most nights instead of cooking and she was too tired to do very much in the way of exercise. Joan told herself that she wasn't actually overweight, just a few pounds heavier than she'd like to be. One day, Joan went to the supermarket and saw that Diabetes UK had a stall outside. After talking to them she found she was at increased risk of developing Type 2 diabetes because her mother had the condition. This was the wake-up call Joan needed to start eating more healthily and begin using an exercise bike in front of the television for twenty minutes every evening. This helped her lose the weight she had gained, plus a bit extra. Joan found she actually enjoyed the exercise as she felt much better, so she made this part of her lifestyle.

Case study: Ruth

Ruth Fairfax had always considered herself healthy. When she was 28, she had her first baby and developed gestational diabetes. She was told that her baby would be large because of her increased BG levels. When Ruth's baby, Sarah, was born she weighed 5.4kg. When Sarah was 18 years old, she developed Type 1 diabetes. She already had an over-active thyroid gland and Sarah's consultant told her that both conditions occurred because her own immune system was attacking healthy tissue in her body. Her mother, Ruth, had developed Type 2 diabetes thirteen years after having Sarah – she had been at increased risk because of her gestational diabetes. Ruth's parents also developed Type 2 diabetes within a year of one another because they were elderly and much less active. Ruth was shocked to realise that three generations of her family had diabetes owing to different causes.

FACT: **Obese men are at higher risk of developing Type 2 diabetes and dangerous levels of liver fats than women.**

Your local government health website helps you assess your risk of developing Type 2 diabetes in two minutes by entering your height, weight and waistline measurement. You can also find out about healthy eating and how to fit more physical activity into your lifestyle. Because the advice is the same across all areas of the country, and in case you can't find this information, the web address for my local area, which you can use to access this information is: medway.gov.uk/diabetes.

Common myths and misconceptions

There are lots of myths about diabetes and many misunderstandings. I once found an Internet website set up for parents of children with Type 1 diabetes that stated that this condition is caused by children eating too many sweets. I was shocked and annoyed, so I contacted them and gave them more accurate information about what causes Type 1 diabetes. After I got in touch, the website disappeared from the Internet.

The world is filled with misinformation – perhaps because over time ideas change, new understandings form, and science separates the truth from the fiction. Here are some more myths I'm keen to bust:

Myth 1: stress causes diabetes

If the body is struggling to maintain BG levels – a stage known as pre-diabetes – excessive stress may cause full-blown diabetes to develop earlier. The hormones released when you are stressed, once you already have diabetes, cause your BG to go up by increasing the amount of glucose that's available to the muscles.

If you already have diabetes, acute stress – say, if you've had an argument with someone – causes an excess of glucose that your body can't deal with. If you suffer from prolonged (chronic) stress, it is a good idea to check your BG more often as you may need to increase your insulin; or if you have Type 2 diabetes and are not prescribed insulin, speak to your GP or diabetes nurse so they can adjust your medication.

Myth 2: having diabetes means you can't eat sweet things

There are times, such as when your BG is low, that you need to eat something sweet in order to bring your BG back up to a normal level. This does not mean you should use your need to avoid *hypoglycaemia* (low BG levels) as an excuse to eat sweet things. I've known several people who keep sweets in their desks at work for 'emergencies', but in fact dip into them all day long.

If you have Type 2 diabetes and take tablets, or use diet and exercise to lower your BG, you have less opportunity to bring your glucose level down again if you eat something sweet for pleasure than if you take insulin.

Medical professionals suggest that for those with Type 1 diabetes, insulin dosages should be given for the carbohydrate content of the food you eat. This is known as Dose Adjustment For Normal Eating, or DAFNE for short. I will go into more detail later, but the good news is if you eat a couple of biscuits containing, for example, 50g of carbohydrate, as long as you give yourself the right amount of insulin to cover the carbohydrate, you can manage your Type 1 diabetes well once you've been on the DAFNE course.

Myth 3: every time you have a hypo, some brain cells die off

Hypoglycaemia is a lack of glucose to fuel the brain and muscles so, unsurprisingly, you can feel tired, shaky and very confused, often with a major lasting headache as a result. Mild to moderate hypos, where you can eat or drink something sweet to reverse it yourself, are not harmful to the brain.

Severe hypos that may lead to unconsciousness or, in some cases, fitting, require the assistance of another person to give an injection of *glucagen*. Glucagen is the same as the glucose stored in the liver and it works very quickly to increase BG, bringing the individual out of unconsciousness (although you'll still feel very delicate). Brain scans following these very severe events have shown some loss of cells. However, the brain is very good at compensating for any loss and rapidly develops new connections so any long-term effect on mental function is minimal.

Myth 4: you can achieve perfect control of blood glucose levels

There is no such thing as perfect glucose control – if you had it, you wouldn't have diabetes because your body would be able to keep BG levels within normal limits on its own. Health professionals – your GP, Practice Nurse, diabetes consultant and diabetes nurse – like you to aim for **normal** to **good** control, although this is not always easy if you have repeated infections and/or *depression*, or *brittle diabetes* – diabetes that is very difficult to control.

Normal to good control means achieving BG readings of between 5.0 and 8.3 mmol/L so the amount of glucose that sticks to your red blood cells over a three-month period – your *HbA1c* or haemoglobin A1c measurement – is between 5.0 and 7.0 per cent (31–53 mmol/L). **Fair** control is a result between 7.0 and 8.0 per cent (53–64 mmol/L); and **poor** control is a result of 9.0 per cent (75 mmol/L) and upwards. In the USA, your HbA1c is known as the *eAG*, or average blood glucose, and this is expressed as a percentage. However, an HbA1c measurement does not record highs and lows, as in your day-to-day blood tests for diabetes management. A result in the good range is highly motivating and proves that you are doing a great job.

FACT: The occasional high or low BG level is to be expected so don't let it throw you. Continue to manage your diabetes as you have been taught and you will be taking control of your condition.

Myth 5: having to take insulin for Type 2 diabetes means you've messed up

Metformin tablets, prescribed to lower BG levels when a person has Type 2 diabetes, may work in this capacity only for a limited number of years before their effectiveness reduces. When this happens, insulin injections are necessary to control BG levels instead. This is not a failure, but the next necessary stage in the effective treatment of Type 2 diabetes.

Taking insulin does mean there is more likelihood of having a low BG, so you will need to do more blood tests each day. The upside of this is that you will feel better as your BG control improves. Sometimes insulin is needed only temporarily because other illnesses stop BG-lowering tablets from working properly. It is also the case that newer medications for Type 2 actually work better than insulin. People taking insulin can be switched to one of these if Metformin stops working and insulin is started as an alternative.

Case study: Kenny

Kenny Walker found his Type 2 diabetes difficult to control. He weighed 89kg, took 65 units of insulin daily and had an HbA1c level of 8.0 per cent (65 mmol/L). His diabetes consultant decided to try Rosiglitazone to help Kenny's BG control. The consultant slowly introduced the medication while lowering Kenny's daily amount of insulin. Six months later, Kenny was delighted to be told that he no longer needed to take insulin: he'd also lost nearly 13kg in weight and his HbA1c level had come down to 6.5 per cent (48 mmol/L).

Another point worth mentioning about Type 2 diabetes and insulin is that, for elderly people, the focus is **not** on the prevention of long-term complications such as eye and kidney disease, which arise over a number of years owing to continually elevated BG levels. Not having to worry about complications simplifies diabetes management considerably.

Myth 6: people with diabetes can't exercise because they'll have a hypo

Any physical effort burns glucose in the muscles, so anything from ironing to hoovering or decorating will have an effect on your BG. The same goes for intense exercise – just ask former Olympic rower, Steve Redgrave, who has Type 1 diabetes. Intense activity can actually raise BG levels because the liver releases stored glucose to power the muscles. The key is **anticipating** glucose needs or potential BG increases and managing them so you don't get caught out.

Although it may seem like the most effort out of all the things people with diabetes are told they should be doing, moderate but regular exercise is a very good way to manage BG levels so they do not creep up. However, certain types of exercise in certain circumstances, like bouncing on a trampoline if you're susceptible to bleeds from the small blood vessels at the back of the eyes (diabetic *retinopathy*), are inadvisable. And those with diabetic *neuropathy* – nerve damage in the feet – and those who are over forty with diabetes should seek medical advice before beginning an exercise programme. Your doctor will advise that you start slowly and build up muscle strength, so don't go too mad too soon!

Case study: Peter

Peter Dawson was 54 with Type 2 diabetes when he decided to buy a treadmill and get fit. He did not tell his GP what he was planning, although the GP had advised Peter to take regular exercise to help manage his BG levels. After the machine was delivered to Peter's home, he found the heavy exercise equipment strenuous to unpack, assemble, and drag into position where he wanted to use it. He then got onto the machine, set the pace button and began running without having exercised for many years. He had sudden pains in his chest and suffered a mild heart attack. His wife, Glynis, called an ambulance and once Peter had undergone tests in hospital, it was discovered that one of his coronary arteries was very narrow. He underwent treatment and has since been properly advised about appropriate exercise. Now when Peter uses his treadmill it is on a much lower setting. He is now doing well.

Myth 7: people with diabetes shouldn't drive

If you have diabetes, check your BG levels before you set out. This is very important and I cannot stress enough that you must stop on long journeys to make sure your BG is not too low and not affecting your judgement: 6.5 mmol/L and above suits me. The Driver and Vehicle Licensing Authority (DVLA) have to be informed if you develop Type 1 diabetes, or if you take insulin temporarily and have had a hypo. They must be told if there are any changes to your treatment or condition, such as numbness in the feet or sight complications. The DVLA will ask you to complete a questionnaire and have eye tests done to measure reaction times and peripheral vision every one, two or three years. There is one driving restriction: the DVLA does not allow people with Type 1 diabetes to drive a Large Goods Vehicle (*LGV*) or a Passenger Carrying Vehicle (*PCV*).

If you treat your diabetes with diet, or diet and tablets, you can hold a licence to drive an LGV or PCV. If you are not prescribed insulin you **do not** have to inform the DVLA about Type 2 diabetes, providing you have necessary eye checks and don't have hypos. You do need to tell them, though, if you have had a hypo in the last year and you needed the assistance of another person to treat it, or if you have reduced or absent hypo warning signs – *hypoglycaemic unawareness* – meaning you know your glucose level only by testing it rather than having any physical symptoms of low BG. In the USA, driving laws for people with diabetes are different in every state and the American Diabetes Association provides details of these.

Myth 8: mung beans and red cabbage can cure diabetes

It is not surprising that people with diabetes want it to go away with as little effort as possible – I certainly do! There are any number of claims in the press and on the Internet about alternative therapies. Unless you are reading the Diabetes UK or American Diabetes Association websites, treat with caution anything you read about diabetes on the Internet, especially when it comes to suggestions that certain foods or products will cure your condition.

I advise that you trust only legitimate sources of information and tried-and-tested treatments provided by your diabetes healthcare team. Your GP may advise you to take aspirin to thin your blood if you have diabetes, aiming to prevent blood clots forming in blood vessels. You may also choose to take the pure herbal supplement *ginkgo biloba*, which we know can improve blood flow to the hands and feet. Other than that, though, sadly there is nothing you can take instead of insulin or your BG-lowering medication.

Chapter 4

A Rollercoaster Of Emotions

'I just felt like my body had let me down big-time…'

Everyone reacts differently to a diagnosis of diabetes – some will react with total shock, others will respond calmly, knowing that the condition can be perfectly manageable. Your own feelings about having diabetes will change over time as you begin to make sense of things and understand what having diabetes means and what you must do. There will almost certainly also be times when it gets too much and you're just fed-up with it all. It's common to feel anger and stress when managing your diabetes, and at the beginning when you've just been diagnosed, you may even try to ignore your condition.

Denial

Developing a serious health condition like diabetes can be like suffering a bereavement because it is the loss of your health. Anger, denial, depression and then finally acceptance are all similar to the pattern of grief. This process can take a very long time – but diabetes doesn't give you that time. As soon as you have a diagnosis, there are all sorts of things you have to do and people you have to see.

Case study: Amy

Amy Parker was 20 when she was diagnosed with Type 1 diabetes. She was also told that for the rest of her life she would need to watch what she was eating and drinking, vigilantly counting carbohydrates and measuring insulin dosages. She would need to do regular BG tests – more if she took exercise – and to take more insulin when she was ill to prevent hyperglycaemia (high BG levels). Her clinic sent her on various carbohydrate-counting and diabetes self-management courses. Amy went into denial and four months after her diagnosis, she was admitted to hospital with dangerously high BG levels which led to *ketoacidosis* – a medical emergency. She was so overwhelmed by the massive change in her life, she felt she couldn't cope. Amy just wanted it all to go away.

Case study: Ravi

Ravi Patel was told he had Type 2 diabetes when he was 44. He was in total shock and refused to believe the diagnosis because he hadn't been feeling ill. Before he'd even come to terms with the news, Ravi's GP arranged for him to attend a DESMOND (Diabetes Education and Self-Management for Ongoing and Newly Diagnosed) education course for people with Type 2. Ravi went along to the course, but he felt that he couldn't take in all the information. Unfortunately, Ravi only went to part of the course. He refused to accept that he would have to cut down on carbohydrate-rich foods and he didn't take the BG-lowering medication prescribed to him. He still has great trouble accepting the diagnosis.

Either of these scenarios may sound familiar. Perhaps you find that even though you do all you can to manage your diabetes, BG levels are still not what both you and your healthcare team are aiming for, so you just feel like giving up. Emotions play a huge role in BG fluctuations. Every person with diabetes experiences times when trying to manage this demanding condition day in, day out becomes all too much. This is normal but not desirable in the long term, especially if other factors, such as depression, exacerbate the situation. Diabetes and depression often go hand in hand and it's common to feel depressed after you have been diagnosed.

FACT: Women with Type 2 diabetes are twice as likely as men with the condition to suffer from depression because of issues such as bodyweight and chronic complications.

You may feel that diabetes is a barrier to doing the things you want to do or being who you want to be, but this is absolutely not the case. Theresa May (the UK's Prime Minister at the time of writing) has Type 1 diabetes, as does ex-professional footballer Gary Mabbutt, and writer Anne Rice, to name a few.

The list of famous people – past and present – with Type 2 diabetes is even longer and includes the likes of Elvis Presley; writers H.G. Wells and Ernest Hemmingway; the hugely successful film director, producer and screen writer George Lucas; and the Oscar-winning actor Tom Hanks. Actress Halle Berry was initially diagnosed with Type 1 diabetes but it was then discovered that she actually has Type 2. The huge number of celebrities and famous people with diabetes goes to show that having the condition is certainly no barrier to achievement.

You may think that despite being given lots of information following your diagnosis, you don't know enough to be able to make alterations to your insulin regime for different situations in life. This is to be expected as you adjust to doing new things and coping with, for example, your first low BG level. Fear of change, and a sense of loss for the life you had before diabetes, is also completely normal.

BLAMING YOURSELF FOR YOUR DIABETES

It is very common to feel you have diabetes because of something you've done or not done. Guilt is especially common for parents if a child develops diabetes. There is absolutely no way to prevent a diagnosis of Type 1 diabetes in either yourself or your child. Equally, with a diagnosis of Type 2 diabetes, blaming yourself is a normal reaction, especially when you feel you haven't, perhaps, looked after yourself very well with a healthy diet or taking regular exercise.

It is true that being overweight, taking little or no exercise and smoking all contribute to poorer health, but you can make big improvements in your management and the effects of Type 2 diabetes on your heart if you eat healthier foods, take exercise several times a week and quit smoking. Self-blame can lead to guilt and depression, but your focus should be on being as healthy as you can be. Blame may also stop you accepting that you have diabetes, or you may accept you have the condition and then blame yourself for causing it.

FACT: **Gaining an understanding of your diabetes and why it happened can give the condition meaning, helping you to cope and adapt to your diagnosis.**

ANXIETY

After you're told you have diabetes, it's common to feel anxious as you come to terms with the diagnosis and learn how to take charge of it. You may also have been feeling anxious *before* your diabetes was diagnosed because you had felt unwell for a while. You may have had concerns over certain symptoms, but just hoped that they would go away. Anxiety also increases in association with going to your doctor, waiting for an appointment, test results and an answer to why you haven't felt right.

> **FACT: People with diabetes who are anxious tend to have higher BG results.**

It's also natural to feel anxious because you expect to have to face lots of life-style changes once you know you have diabetes. This can be associated with the condition itself; your treatment and having to remember to take it on time; your BG results and whether they are too high or too low; needing to rely on health professionals to advise you; or lacking the information and support that you need. These anxieties should become fewer as you learn to cope with your condition. Unfortunately, if your BG control is not good, you may become anxious about how this will affect you over time, and about developing chronic complications of diabetes, especially if you have symptoms such as tingling in your feet, or blurred vision.

Case study: Peter

Peter McKechnie developed Type 1 diabetes when he was 25. Peter resented his condition and begrudgingly did the absolute minimum to manage it by giving himself insulin twice a day and only testing his BG before bed. He was incredibly anxious about how having diabetes would affect his life: his future job prospects; travelling and going on holiday with his friends; whether he'd develop sight complications that would stop him driving; and needing to rely on other people if he had a serious hypo. Peter discussed these issues with a counsellor who was trained in helping people with chronic medical conditions and he eventually came to realise that he needed to take responsibility for his diabetes and to manage it as well as possible. This was because all the issues Peter was anxious about were more likely to happen if he had poor BG control, increasing his risk of complications and problems associated with his diabetes.

ANGER

The majority of people with long-term – chronic – medical conditions feel angry, especially when it's a condition like diabetes that needs a great deal of self-care. Experts agree that anger comes from a build-up of physical energy – stress – that needs to be released from the body. Anger is triggered by frustration, tension, hostility and irritation, and the way you cope with it is the key to stopping anger from damaging your health. Anger at a situation or another person creates negative thoughts because of *your perception* of that situation or that person's actions. As with all negative thoughts, it is a good idea to try and think through why they are in your mind and bothering you, and the same is true of angry emotions. You may not realise it, but there are three different kinds of anger[1]:

- RAGE is explosive, violent, uncontrolled anger expressed as a destructive force.
- RESENTMENT is internal anger that boils away and is not unleashed on the person or situation that's making you angry. It can bubble away for some time making you feel ill at ease, and this is damaging both physically and mentally.
- INDIGNATION is a more controlled form of anger, such as saying, 'How dare you!' to someone so they know they've overstepped the mark. It's far less damaging and perhaps the most positive form of anger.

When you're angry, you don't stop to think about what form your anger should take as it's a defensive, reactionary emotion. You feel anger because someone or something has hurt you. Being diagnosed with diabetes can certainly cause anger for lots of reasons[2]:

1   Clark, M. (2004a), *Understanding Diabetes* (West Sussex, England: John Wiley & Sons Ltd.), pp.38–9.
2   Jarvis, S. & Rubin, A. (2003), *Diabetes for Dummies* (Chichester: John Wiley & Sons Ltd.), p.14.

- Your body has let you down.
- You now have a chronic medical condition.
- You have to look after diabetes as though it were a demanding child.
- You have to monitor what you eat and drink.
- You feel your diabetes stops you doing what you want to do.
- Your family and friends don't understand diabetes or they make comments about you not looking after yourself properly.
- You can't manage your diabetes well, even though you try really hard.

What triggers your anger is a personal thing, but if you often feel angry, it's worth thinking about how to deal with it.

How do I deal with anger?

Find a physical release[3], and by that I don't mean punching someone, however much satisfaction it might bring! Knowing that you *have a choice* is important. You can throw a tantrum in the supermarket over the fact that someone just ran over your foot with their trolley, or you can view the situation as an accident, be calm and accept that there's nothing you can do about it. Hopefully the person will apologise, but if they don't and burning resentment seethes through your whole body, *stay in control* and congratulate yourself for not losing your rag in public.

Exercise is a great way to reduce stress and anger so that you don't have to get physically involved in the fight! If the anger-inducing situation has also made you very sad, a good cry can release the tension and the anger, and you will feel much better afterwards. Anger may also be controlled by labelling it as a person, so when you feel angry you say to yourself, 'Here's [insert a suitable name!] here to irritate and annoy me.' Other methods are counting out loud or shouting a word you have decided is your anger-word. People may stare, but it's better than shouting something far worse!

3   Clark, M. (2004a), *Understanding Diabetes* (West Sussex, England: John Wiley & Sons Ltd.), p.41.

GUILT

Another strong emotion associated with the diagnosis of any health issue is that of guilt. This is especially related to thoughts of not having looked after yourself properly, or having done something wrong. Guilt also pops up every time you don't feel like exercising, or if you realise you forgot to inject insulin or take glucose-reducing tablets at a certain time. Be assured – everyone with diabetes has done this at one time or another!

Feeling guilty is a negative emotion that can make diabetes self-management more difficult. Guilt is based on a feeling of unease owing to bad behaviour – because you feel you've done something wrong or you should have done something differently[4]. It's also the feeling you get when you've been blaming yourself – for example, if you eat something 'naughty'. The guilt if you eat a cake is normal, but believing you are a bad person for doing so is negative and destructive.

When you have diabetes, you may feel guilty because you feel you could have prevented it in some way; or have prevented some of the complications of diabetes. Guilt also raises its head when you don't look after yourself as well as you know you should. It is completely *normal* to feel guilty about aspects of diabetes and its care.

Case study: Katriona

Katriona Billings had great difficulty overcoming her sense of guilt when she developed Type 1 diabetes. She also had asthma and she'd read that the medication in her inhaler caused the pancreas to release insulin, so she wondered if she'd taken too much of it, triggering her diabetes. Her feelings of guilt were so strong that she found them exhausting. She also felt guilty for the worry and the

4   Clark, M. (2004a), *Understanding Diabetes* (West Sussex, England: John Wiley & Sons Ltd.), p.42.

burden she imagined she had put on her family and for resenting her happy, carefree friends who had no idea about diabetes or how it affected someone's life. When Katriona realised why she felt guilty, she was able to challenge the emotion and recognise that her diabetes was not her fault, and nor was it the fault of other people. She also realised that there was little point in feeling angry that other people didn't understand the condition. Katriona now has more positive energy to spend on managing her diabetes than feeling guilty about it.

There are ways of dealing with feelings of guilt so that this emotion is easier to deal with. M. Clark suggests the following:

How can I deal with my feelings of guilt?

- Focus on *why* you have feelings of guilt. Is it, for example, something you did or didn't do, or something someone else did that you know about and feel is wrong? Isolating the reason for guilt can make the situation feel less of a burden, or even make it go away completely.
- If possible, share how you feel about your diabetes with others who are involved, and try to come up with a solution to overcoming those feelings. This might not be appropriate to your specific situation, but if it is you can begin to think in a more positive way and you'll feel less guilty.
- Don't cover up or try to ignore guilt that you feel you can't cope with as this will make it worse. It's also wise to avoid drinking and smoking more, or binge eating to try and take your mind off the guilt rather than facing it.
- Once you've identified the problem (let's say you often eat sweets when you know you shouldn't) and a potential way to deal with it, contact a health professional who can offer you appropriate support and won't judge you. This might be your GP, Practice Nurse or diabetes nurse.

Stress

The word 'stress' can be used to mean anything from dealing with a difficult situation to the body's physical and mental reaction to everyday demands. We have to adapt ourselves to the situations we find ourselves in every day, whether that's a workman outside your house with a pneumatic drill; travelling on a very crowded train to work; or the stress involved in taking an exam or moving house. Whatever the trigger, stress causes a physical reaction (sweaty palms, heart palpitations, a headache, and/or diarrhoea, tightness in the throat, and tension or nausea) as well as an emotional one (irritation, bad temper, anxiety, unease, worry, panic, anger or frustration).

How does stress affect my diabetes?

When you're stressed and you have diabetes, the physical changes the body makes to deal with that stress – releasing glucose to the muscles in the fight-or-flight response, and adrenaline to make sure we're alert – increases BG levels. This is harmful if you can't burn off this excess glucose or reduce it with insulin. Other reactions to stress making your diabetes difficult to control are:

- An increase in blood flow to your muscles – taking glucose there to fuel them – which increases your blood pressure.
- Blood vessels are made smaller, increasing your heart rate, and breathing becomes rapid to supply more oxygen to all parts of the body.
- Slowed digestion as blood is taken away from breaking down food and diverted to the muscles.
- Shaking and sweating, like the symptoms of having a hypo. You may feel an adrenaline rush hurrying through your system, and a headache may develop.
- Dry mouth and nausea.
- Cramped, tight muscles.

If you can't actually take your frustration out on the object causing you stress, or run away from something that is bothering you, then the stress isn't released and it has no purpose in, or outlet from the body. Accumulated and prolonged stress can severely affect the immune system so that serious illness occurs.

FACT: Prolonged, harmful imbalance in the body caused by stress can lead to heart disease, hardening of the arteries, Type 2 diabetes and certain types of cancer.

When stress affects us, stored glucose released into the bloodstream increases BG, requiring more insulin or BG-lowering medication. The increase in BG may also go undetected when you are stressed because you're preoccupied with the situation rather than regularly checking your BG levels. You also may not want to, or have time to eat or exercise, or you may choose to deal with the stress by drinking alcohol or smoking more than you usually do. You don't need me to tell you that these ways of 'coping' aren't particularly healthy ways of dealing with stress.

How can I deal with stress?

As you can see from the ways stress affects the body, you need to deal with stress so that you're in control of your diabetes. There are several ways to help overcome the effects of stress on the body but you need to keep in mind[5]:

FACT: You can manage and control stress, but you can't completely remove it.

---

5   Clark, M. (2004a), *Understanding Diabetes* (West Sussex, England: John Wiley & Sons Ltd.), p.47.

- Use relaxation techniques such as deep breathing, meditation and hypnosis to reduce stress. These are effective because they allow your body to rest, especially if you haven't been sleeping well. They will also help you feel calmer and in control of the situation and of your diabetes, increasing your sense of wellbeing. Before you go to sleep, try a visualisation to help you feel calm and stress-free. Use all your senses. For example, imagine walking in a beautiful garden, planted with colourful and wonderfully scented flowers and that you hear a waterfall nearby. This sort of imagery, if practised regularly, really can help reduce stress.

- Identify why you are feeling stressed. Knowing what the exact cause is – for example, trying to fit BG testing into a very busy lifestyle – can help you to devise ways of dealing with it. Telling yourself you are just too busy to manage your diabetes during the day isn't specific enough – you need to know what the problem is to find a solution and reduce the stress.

- When you know what the problem is, the next thing to think about is how you react to that problem. Reacting before you've fully assessed the situation can mean that things are not as bad in reality. Once you recognise you're doing this, you can take a breath when a stressful situation happens before allowing your emotions to overwhelm you.

Deal with things that stress you by breaking them down into manageable parts so they don't seem such a big deal. Identify whether you tend to react to stress physically (shouting and screaming), or emotionally (worrying and internalising). When you know why and how you react, you can alter this response and, over time with repetition, your brain will automatically react in the way you want it to.

- Stay away from things that cause you stress as much as possible. Obviously, if it's having diabetes itself that stresses you, then you need to discuss better coping strategies with your diabetes team. If you can't avoid what stresses you, change the way you react. Don't say or think, 'I knew this would happen to me, it always does', or, 'I bet no one else has these problems'; instead try 'This has happened, but I can overcome it by…' or 'I'm going to call X, as I know they can help me through this.'

- Exercise is not only a good way of reducing your BG levels, it also helps to relieve stress. The best exercise is enjoyable exercise.
- Take up a hobby or leisure activity. It's a diversion and stops you thinking about the situation. If it's a productive hobby, the creation of something new can be motivating and is also very therapeutic.
- Try to get into a regular sleep pattern, going to bed and getting up at regular times each day so that your body clock is stable and you get good amounts of rest.

Fear

It is completely natural to be fearful when you're told you have diabetes, and for what lies ahead. You may not think of questions to ask about diabetes until after the news has sunk in, or feel you can't ask something because it seems like a silly question. All the issues surrounding diabetes as a chronic condition can lead to fear of the unknown.

FACT: Between 4 and 10 per cent of people with and without diabetes have a fear of needles.

If you take insulin to treat your diabetes, having a fear of needles can make this difficult. There are options available if this applies to you so you can inject without seeing the needle. Many people say that it's a fear of what's going to happen rather than the actual process or any pain that might happen at the time. *Insulin pump therapy* – where a small plastic tube, or *cannula*, is placed under the skin to deliver insulin as required – is also an option for people with needle phobia. This is especially helpful if you currently have to take *multiple daily injections*. Your diabetes team will be able to arrange this if appropriate, or show you how to inject insulin as quickly and painlessly as possible.

When you have had diabetes for a little while, the questions you have may be answered in the course of time, but this doesn't mean that the fear goes away. For example, you may worry about 'Will I develop complications?' (such as eye and kidney disease) for many years. If complications do develop, then fear of how they will progress can take over. I think that's because the possibility of complications is drummed into us from diagnosis. This type of fear is to be expected, but living in a permanent state of fearfulness is not healthy for you or your diabetes.

FACT: **The best way to overcome a fear of complications is to control your diabetes as well as you possibly can to keep BG levels within normal limits.**

The way to deal with diabetes-related fear is to plan for situations *before* they happen. Below are some ways to overcome general fears associated with your diabetes[6]:

- You may fear that you won't be able to cope with having diabetes because it's too difficult and that potential problems will be impossible to overcome. The best way to deal with this is to write down the things that you fear about diabetes self-management and then find solutions, such as speaking to your diabetes nurse.
- If you fear night-time hypos and have reduced hypo awareness and you live alone, it may be appropriate to ask your diabetes nurse about using insulin pump therapy and continual glucose monitoring to ensure your BG remains at a safe limit during sleep.

6   Clark, M. (2004a), *Understanding Diabetes* (West Sussex, England: John Wiley & Sons Ltd.), p.50.

- Remind yourself that chronic complications are not inevitable when you have diabetes. If, over time, you do develop *mild* neuropathy – nerve damage – in your feet, mild *nephropathy* in your kidneys, or mild retinopathy in your eyes, the effects are not severe and you can still live your life the way you want to.
- Use the fear of complications to motivate you to manage your diabetes in the best way you can to keep your HbA1c levels – the glucose sticking to the red blood cells – low.
- If you have had diabetes for a number of years and you have complications that now limit you, concentrate on the things you can still do. You may not, for example, be able to drive any more because of sight problems but you may be able to draw or paint.
- Don't dwell on feeling like you're a burden to your family and friends when you need some help with daily tasks because of long-term complications. The people closest to you like to be involved in helping you with your diabetes as it makes them feel needed and useful!
- You may fear pain in relation to complications. *Peripheral neuropathy* – burning and needle-like sensations in the feet or hands – can be painful, but there are medications that can treat this – *Gabapentin*. Other complications, such as autonomic neuropathy – damage to the nerves controlling functions like digestion and heartbeat; diabetic nephropathy and retinopathy **are not** painful conditions. Everyone with diabetes, as with the non-diabetic population, gets a twinge of pain now and then so try not to fear that something serious is going on with your diabetes.
- Some people fear how other people will react – are you worried about telling people you have diabetes? So many people have the condition now – one in four – that it's not something to worry about. Diabetes isn't something you can catch, so people won't avoid you if you tell them. The response I usually get is, 'Oh, my mother or father or sister or brother or son or daughter or aunty or uncle has that!' or even, 'So do I!'
- If you feel that you have to tell someone important about your

diabetes and you fear how he/she may react, try to prepare answers to any anticipated questions beforehand.

FACT: You don't have to tell an employer that you have dia- betes unless they ask any medical questions, but you may want to tell them anyway so they know what to do if you have a hypo at work.

- Don't fear travelling to other countries if you have diabetes. It's such a common condition globally now that hospitals, clinics and pharmacies will be aware of what you need if you become ill, or run out of your medication. If you fear that you don't speak the language of the country you're visiting, simply make sure you have a phrase book with you, or use the Internet to work out some key phrases before you leave, write them down and carry them with you – you can show them to a pharmacist or doctor, if that's easier.
- Plan your trip carefully and make sure you take extra medication and supplies with you. If it's a hot country you are visiting, buy a cooler bag for your insulin as **heat degrades insulin** (it's a protein) – think of how cheese changes when you grill it. Check on the Internet or with your travel agent before you depart to find out where the nearest medical facilities are to where you'll be staying to give you some peace of mind.

FACT: By facing the things about diabetes that you're afraid of, whether physically overcoming them or mentally identifying them, you can reduce and even get rid of the fear.

Case study: Mauro

Mauro Pelargrino was told he had Type 2 diabetes after having a routine blood test at his GP surgery. He felt alone and isolated, but most of all he felt fear. His GP suggested he go along to a local diabetes support group where he could meet and speak to other people with the condition and discuss how he felt. Mauro didn't really want to go along and sit in a room full of people with diabetes because he felt they wouldn't understand his fear, and that they would all be old hands at managing the condition. After Mauro had been to a few meetings he realised that everyone else was struggling with the same issues as he was, and he admits he learned lots of ways to help himself to manage his diabetes.

COPING STRATEGIES

Case study: Ana

Ana Blake was shocked when she was first told that she had Type 2 diabetes but she quickly realised that this was something she needed to get on top of. She read as much as she could about how to manage the condition because she was curious, and found that this actually helped her to accept her diagnosis and begin to manage it properly. Diabetes wasn't something that she wanted in her life, but Ana realised that she had to face up to the news, or else the situation would become worse.

Coping with the diagnosis of any chronic condition is similar to coping with a very stressful event because we must adapt and deal with a long-term negative change in lifestyle that wasn't expected, wanted or planned for[7]. If the way you usually cope with stressful events is to try and ignore them, this won't work with diabetes as it will cause you more problems in the long run.

Other reactions that some people have are blaming someone else for their diabetes, treating it as though it's not a big deal, and letting the diagnosis wash over them without responding to what they're told. These forms of 'coping' result in poor BG control. Those people who take the news seriously but don't react with distress tend to deal with the management of their diabetes very well.

RELIEF

Many people are actually relieved when they finally get a diagnosis and an explanation of their symptoms, especially if they knew something was wrong, but didn't know what. As we've already seen, the symptoms of diabetes can be very different from person to person. For this reason, knowing that diabetes is the cause helps provide hope that insulin or BG-reducing medication will control these symptoms and improve wellbeing.

Case study: Andy

Andy Cowling was 60 and had been feeling tired for a long time. He put it down to getting older and perhaps not getting enough iron in his diet, imagining that he might be anaemic. Andy bought himself some iron supplements from the chemist, but after three months, there was no improvement and he still felt tired. Andy then thought he must be imagining feeling tired because it was to

---

7   Clark, M. (2004a), *Understanding Diabetes* (West Sussex, England: John Wiley & Sons Ltd.), p.32.

be expected in a man of his age – needing a nap mid-afternoon and a second cup of tea after each meal as his mouth was dry. This went on for a year until, finally, Andy had to go to the dentist and she told him that he should visit his GP for a BG test. Andy followed his dentist's advice and discovered that he had Type 2 diabetes a week later. He felt a huge sense of relief when he received the diagnosis, realising that he had a reason for his tiredness and thirst. He also felt daft that he hadn't wanted to make a fuss!

There are people who try to put on a brave face or make excuses for the symptoms of diabetes, claiming that they're owing to the pressures of work, getting older, or even that they're just imagining having to go to the toilet more often because they're drinking more cups of tea every day. This is a form of denial and it acts as a protection measure rather than admitting that there is something wrong. Finding out that there is a genuine physical reason for the symptoms helps the individual realise it wasn't 'all in their head'.

CHANGING MOODS AND EMOTIONS

How you feel can be down to your BG being too low or too high: mood swings are also very normal in people with diabetes because of this. Your brain needs a constant supply of glucose to function properly, so if your BG is low, you become irritable, sad, tired, short-tempered and upset. The effects of high and low BG on the brain appear as very similar symptoms and sometimes testing your BG is the only way to find out. You may not even connect being angry or irritated with your BG – it took me some years to recognise this as I just thought I had little patience! Having a high level of available glucose does not make your brain work better: it actually irritates it because too much glucose is a toxin.

Case study: Sally

Sally Morris had Type 1 diabetes that was very difficult to control, meaning that her BG levels would swing from high to low without warning – something she found hard to cope with. Her husband, Gary, was used to this situation and didn't take the things Sally said to heart, such as her shouting that he should leave her alone when he was trying to help reverse her hypoglycaemia with sweet tea. Gary would assure Sally that her moods were not her fault. One day, Gary's parents came to stay and Sally had a bad hypo followed by prolonged hyperglycaemia because her liver had released stored glucose – Sally was battling to reduce it. Gary's parents didn't understand the situation and had never seen Sally act in this 'snappy and sarcastic' way before. Sally later overheard her mother-in-law describing her as hostile. This upset Sally greatly and she was overwhelmed with a sense that people just didn't understand. She decided to apologise, although she strongly felt she shouldn't have to. When she said sorry, she expected her parents-in-law to understand that it was her BG levels but instead they said, 'We don't know why you had to act like that.' Sally was angry at the injustice for a long while afterwards and felt isolated by the experience.

High BG levels make you feel irritated, on edge, frustrated, annoyed and even vicious. You may say horrible things to other people and, not withstanding how they have to develop a thick skin and understand that you don't mean it, you are left with feelings of guilt afterwards for 'being moody'. It's a difficult one because at some stage, your personality will be temporarily altered by your BG and explaining this to those around you can be hard.

It is perfectly normal to feel overwhelmed by a diagnosis of diabetes and trying to meet the daily demands necessary to manage the condition well. Many people find they have difficulties with adopting lots of new behaviours into their life – taking insulin or medication in the right dose at the right time, doing regular blood tests throughout the day, weighing or carbohydrate-counting foods, keeping active, attending various hospital clinics and GP checks, and so on. Self-care habits such as these take months, if not longer, to become the sorts of things you do without thinking each day. Think how often you had to be reminded to clean your teeth as a child before you did it automatically!

A much easier way around having to do new self-care tasks is to take one thing at a time. Obviously, some things take priority, such as the need for regular insulin or BG-lowering medication and blood tests, but if you set your own priorities to get to grips with something new that you feel is a realistic goal, it is an achievement when you master it. This also means you are less likely to go back to your old ways. I have, however, known people who say that they sometimes still forget to do their insulin injections after twenty years of having Type 1 diabetes. They realise only when they eat and feel very sick about an hour afterwards because their BG is sky high. This goes to show that even the most experienced person with diabetes can still slip up sometimes. But you learn from it, so you don't do the same thing again.

> **FACT:** The way you feel – mental health – is just as important as physical health.

Understanding how emotions affect your diabetes is the key to coming to terms with the condition and being able to manage these ups and downs so that you are in control of your diabetes rather than it being in control of you. One key way of being in control is developing what is called *self-efficacy* – the self-confidence to do things, like using a BG-testing machine, or drawing up and injecting insulin, and building on that to know you can tackle similar challenges.

I recently had to start using a new *insulin pump* – a piece of technology that delivers insulin continuously under the skin. I had to force myself to get acquainted with it because it was different to what I was used to. It was the same principle as the insulin pumps I'd used for the past eighteen years, but it reminded me that with diabetes, you never stop learning.

Other people can also be very good at making you feel bad unintentionally because they want the best for you. Because diabetes is the only chronic condition where the person who has it provides 95 per cent of their own care, other people's comments can cut deep. Most people are only being kind, even if that comes out as what is actually thoughtlessness.

Case study: Colin

Colin Stoddard was diagnosed with Type 2 diabetes over ten years ago but felt that other people were his biggest problem. It seemed that wherever he went, people assumed they knew more about his condition than he did, or that they were interfering in his life. At work, colleagues would say things like, 'Should you be eating that?' when Colin's BG was low and he was having a biscuit with his morning coffee. At home, his wife would often suggest that he should be walking the dog or gardening to get some exercise, and if he went to his daughter's house for Sunday lunch, she would control Colin's food portions rather than letting him choose for himself. Over the years, these small annoyances built up into major irritations and, in the end, Colin told people that he would make his own decisions, thank you very much. He then felt guilty because he knew everyone was just looking out for him. He just couldn't win!

The more you actively learn about your diabetes, the better. **Take your time and go at your own pace.** I won't lie – it's a steep learning curve, but the more you find out about up-to-date and reliable diabetes information, education and support, the less likely you are to worry: a better understanding means you can manage the condition effectively.

> **FACT:** Feeling diabetes-related guilt is like taking your diabetes medication – it's an integral part of the condition.

DEPRESSION

Although the conditions are physically unconnected, depression and diabetes can run side by side. Depression does develop more often in people with diabetes, and Type 2 diabetes can develop following a period of depression. Both depression and diabetes can be isolating and cause you to think that no one understands or that you just want to give up. This can be the case if you're trying hard to do your best, but your BG levels don't show that. As we've already seen, many things affect your diabetes control, such as stress (which can increase BG owing to hormonal variations that make the liver release stored glucose). Stress may occur as a result of being in denial about your diagnosis and in association with feelings of anger, but it's important not to let this manifest in the form of ignoring the need for insulin or tablets.

> **FACT:** Clinical depression affects at least 15 per cent of people with diabetes and can have an adverse effect on BG control and diabetes self-management and chronic complications in both adults and children.

Case study: Sylvia

Sylvia Walker felt her life was over when she was diagnosed with diabetes. She decided she was no use to anyone and that her efforts to control her Type 2 diabetes were useless. Sylvia felt so low, she wondered why she was even bothering at all as it was 'only Type 2' and, in her eyes, not as serious as the Type 1 diabetes affecting one of her relatives. She reasoned that as her diabetes was causing her to feel so bad psychologically, if she just didn't think about it then maybe her life could go back to the way it was. Sylvia's GP prescribed anti-depressants to try to lift her mood and she is currently waiting to see a counsellor who specialises in depression and health issues.

Depression is three times more likely to occur in people with diabetes and this is a problem because it not only impacts on mental health, it also affects a person's ability to self-manage their condition[8]. This, in turn, leads to poor BG control, which can trigger chronic complications over time.

> **FACT:** Although depression is a major issue for people with diabetes, it is often not diagnosed, especially if the person doesn't tell their GP, Practice Nurse or diabetes team how they feel.

What are the symptoms of depression[9]?

There are many symptoms of depression, such as:

- Feeling very sad, unmotivated or dejected.
- Loss of appetite that is not because of high BG levels or your diabetes medication.
- Being unable to sleep because sad thoughts keep running through your mind.
- Sleeping too much because that way, you can switch off your mind.

---

8 Clark, M. (2004b), 'Identification and treatment of depression in people with diabetes', *Diabetes and Primary Care* 5(3), pp.124–7.
9 Ibid., pp.124–7.

- Withdrawing from the social events you enjoy.
- Crying for no particular reason, especially if this is unlike you.
- Focusing on things that happened in the past that you can do nothing about.
- Feeling hopeless, inadequate or worthless.
- Often feeling angry and very irritable even when it's not because of your BG levels.
- Feeling more fearful of situations.
- Having little interest in work, family or other interests, or lacking concentration.
- Having little energy, but not if this is owing to your BG or other health issues.
- Thinking, speaking or acting in a more reserved way than normal.

The more of these symptoms that you recognise in yourself or another person with diabetes, the more likely you/they are to have depression.

How can I help myself?

The best thing you can do to keep depression at bay, or under control if you already have it, is to make sure your BG levels are within normal limits of 5.0–7.0 mmol/L[10]. This is because hormonal and chemical changes that occur in the body with depression act to increase BG levels and so, even if you don't feel like eating – or haven't eaten anything – your BG may still be very high.

> FACT: Depression interacts negatively with diabetes, leading to unpredictable diabetes control and a 1.8-per-cent increase in HbA1c.

10 Clark, M. (2004a), *Understanding Diabetes* (West Sussex, England: John Wiley & Sons Ltd.), pp.35–8.

There are other things you can do as well as keeping tight control of your BG to help fight depression. Focusing on a long-term goal can really help to reduce depressive symptoms as it takes a lot of effort to be depressed – by diverting your attention, your brain is dealing with reaching your goal and not generating depressive feelings. Similarly, keeping yourself physically active not only helps to reduce your BG, it also helps release anger, irritations and frustrations – if you choose an activity that makes you feel positive – by releasing 'feel-good' hormones (*endorphins*). Don't forget to consult your diabetes team if you think you might be depressed.

FACT: It's important to recognise when you're thinking in a negative way. Ask yourself, what set it off? Can you do something to change the situation, or is it something you have no control over?

FACT: Emotions are constantly changing so what you feel and think isn't lasting. The key is *noticing* your mood so you can know why you're thinking a certain way.

It also helps to remember that everyone has something to worry about in their life, so trying to see things from another person's perspective can help you see why they react in a certain way. Often, we don't know what others have to cope with. Negative thoughts can lead to negative actions.

FACT: Negative thoughts are not good for your diabetes control!

Share your feelings, thoughts and worries with other people who will listen and care – that is, not a random stranger in the doctor's surgery who will shrug their shoulders and make you feel worse. Make sure you tell your diabetes team how you feel as they may be able to refer you to a specialist psychologist or counsellor who can help resolve the issues causing your depression. It may be the case that your depression is caused by a chemical imbalance or deficiency, so if it lasts for a long time, even after treatment with anti-depressant medication or therapy, this may be the reason and it can be treated.

FACT: If someone doesn't like the fact you have diabetes, then you don't need them in your life!

RELATIONSHIPS

Partners and good friends

When you have diabetes, it can be difficult to know when to introduce this into a conversation with a new partner or friend. You may imagine that your new soul mate will go running for the hills if you introduce diabetes into the conversation, and this can make you nervous about telling them and especially, how to explain it.[11]

Most people have heard of diabetes before, but they may not know much about it, other than that it's something to do with sugar. Don't expect people to automatically understand what you're telling them about your diabetes. But if someone is truly interested in you as a person, the fact you have diabetes won't put them off!

11 Clark, M. (2004a), *Understanding Diabetes* (West Sussex, England: John Wiley & Sons Ltd.), p.50.

Case study: Lee

Lee Brown was 19 when he met his girlfriend, Annie. After a few dates, he became more and more worried that telling her he had diabetes would put her off. Lee's mum, Linda, told him he should just explain the facts simply, making sure he mentioned how low BG levels affected him and how Annie could help. When Lee plucked up the courage to let Annie know, he explained the basics of the condition, hypo warning signs and how to treat it quickly. She listened carefully and then asked sensible questions. This made Lee realise that Annie was actually interested in his diabetes – she wanted to know as much as possible. Two years on they are now engaged, have bought a house together and hope to marry later this year.

Don't ever feel that you have to cover up your diabetes: everyone you meet usually has some kind of medical history. In the case of diabetes, it's telling people if you need to eat, do an injection, do a blood test, feel low – whatever. People *do* generally understand and they are usually interested in finding out more. This might annoy the heck out of you, but see it as an opportunity to educate others about what you have to do every day to keep well.

Chapter 5

How Will Diabetes Affect Me?

'I know that managing diabetes is a head-to-toe problem.'

BG levels are continually fluctuating, especially when you eat. This is why you will need to measure your BG levels often throughout the day and sometimes during the night, and even more often if you develop an infection like a cold or flu, or when you exercise. How often you should test your BG is determined by the kind of diabetes you have, the treatment you take for it, and how well that treatment manages your condition to keep it stable. Variations in BG, as we've just seen, can have an enormous effect on personality and mood. This is not something we can control, but trying to keep BG within normal limits allows the brain to function correctly without irritation from high glucose levels, or to go into panic and shock from very low levels.

Hospital blood tests

The blood tests you do yourself at home are the best way of showing you what your BG is at that moment in time and what you need to do next, but they don't tell you how good your overall diabetes self-management is over, say, several months. When you have an HbA1c test done at the hospital or a blood-testing clinic, a sample of blood is taken from a vein to see how much glucose has stuck to your red blood cells over a three-month period. This is because red blood cells are renewed every three months, so you won't be asked to have this test done any more frequently than this while your diabetes is being stabilised and your consultant reviews how well your treatment is working. Once your diabetes is under control, you will usually have an HbA1c blood test once every six months to a year for your annual diabetes review.

It was decided a few years ago to stop measuring HbA1c as a percentage concentration of glucose in the blood over time and to now measure it in millimoles per litre – mmol/L – in the same way that home blood-testing machines do. I personally prefer the old-fashioned percentage measurement of HbA1c as an indicator of how good my BG control has been, as do some diabetes specialists. I've provided a table below to show how HbA1c percentage converts to mmol/L and vice versa, so you can judge how good your glucose control has been. You may also find this table useful if you read books and articles about diabetes published a few years ago that have used percentage HbA1c values.[1]

HbA1c %	mmol/L	HbA1c %	mmol/L	HbA1c %	mmol/L	HbA1c %	mmol/L
4.0	20	6.0	42	8.0	64	10.0	86
4.1	21	6.1	43	8.1	65	10.1	87
4.2	22	6.2	44	8.2	66	10.2	88
4.3	23	6.3	45	8.3	67	10.3	89
4.4	25	6.4	46	8.4	68	10.4	90
4.5	26	6.5	48	8.5	69	10.5	91
4.6	27	6.6	49	8.6	70	10.6	92
4.7	28	6.7	50	8.7	72	10.7	93
4.8	29	6.8	51	8.8	73	10.8	95
4.9	30	6.9	52	8.9	74	10.9	96
5.0	31	7.0	53	9.0	75	11.0	97
5.1	32	7.1	54	9.1	76	11.1	98
5.2	33	7.2	55	9.2	77	11.2	99
5.3	34	7.3	56	9.3	78	11.3	100
5.4	36	7.4	57	9.4	79	11.4	101
5.5	37	7.5	58	9.5	80	11.5	102
5.6	38	7.6	60	9.6	81	11.6	103
5.7	39	7.7	61	9.7	83	11.7	104
5.8	40	7.8	62	9.8	84	11.8	105
5.9	41	7.9	63	9.9	85	11.9	107

1   www.southend.nhs.uk/media/44653/hba1c_conversion_table.pdf

Case study: Angela

Angela White was planning to become pregnant and was advised by her GP to tighten her BG control to make sure she was as healthy as possible before conception. Her HbA1c had been 7.2 per cent (55 mmol/L), but her GP suggested she aim for 6.0–6.5 per cent (42–48 mmol/L). Angela was motivated to test her BG more frequently and to exercise after meals to stop any sharp increases in BG. When she had her next HbA1c test three months later, she had achieved her goal and, by keeping a close eye on her BG levels, she went on to have a healthy pregnancy and a normal-weight baby girl. Because Angela had made the lifestyle changes of exercising after meals and checking her BG often for the sake of her baby and had done this for a year, she kept up the new routine, finding that it had given her more energy.

FACT: Knowing your HbA1c can help you plan to make changes in your diabetes self-management to reduce high glucose levels that make you feel sluggish.

YOUR OWN BG-MONITORING TESTS

The reason you need to check your BG levels regularly is to find out if you have too much or too little insulin or glucose-lowering medication working at certain times of the day and night. If there is too little insulin, your BG levels will be high; too much insulin and your BG will be low.

High blood glucose – hyperglycaemia

HYPERGLYCAEMIA is the medical term for high blood glucose levels. When there is a lack of insulin, or it can't be used properly by the body, high BG levels are the result. As a basic rule, this means glucose-metre readings in double figures. If this situation lasts over a period of time, the excess glucose causes the blood to become acidic and if too little insulin is available, this becomes a medical emergency known as diabetic ketoacidosis – DKA – needing hospital attention. When ketoacidosis happens, your body doesn't have enough insulin or BG-lowering medication to work properly. Instead of being able to use glucose for fuel, when there is not enough insulin, your body has to switch to using fat and protein for energy, meaning your muscle can break down instead. The acid by-products of this breakdown are called *ketones* – hence diabetic ketoacidosis.

FACT: Make sure you do more BG tests when you are ill. Increasing insulin dosages to avoid hyperglycaemia can keep you out of hospital as you will be reducing your risk of diabetic ketoacidosis, but make sure BG isn't becoming too low.

Causes of diabetic ketoacidosis

- Under-dosing or deliberate repeated omission of insulin – your body can't go without insulin for long as it is needed to convert starch and glucose into energy.
- Any kind of infection that increases BG levels so that you need more insulin.
- Physical or emotional trauma.
- Heart attack.
- Alcohol and/or drug abuse, particularly cocaine use.
- Medications such as *corticosteroids* – these come as tablets, inhalers, injections and creams used to treat inflammation – and diuretics (water tablets).

Symptoms of DKA[2]

- Sickness and vomiting – this happens because of the build-up of acids from the breakdown of fat and protein and because your body is lacking certain chemicals.

- Rapid breathing – known as *Kussmaul breathing*. This happens when your blood is very acidic and your body tries to pant out some of this acid. The acidic breath of a person with DKA often smells like acetone – nail polish remover – or pear drops.

- Tiredness and lethargy – this happens because your body can't use glucose for fuel when your BG is very high. Your brain cannot work as normal with thick, syrupy blood lacking in essential nutrients when you have ketoacidosis.

- Weakness in the muscles – again, this happens because your body can't use glucose as fuel for muscle function; instead the body begins to break down fat and then protein in the muscles instead.

Case study: Michael

Michael Barlow was 18, had Type 1 diabetes and was always getting colds and sore throats because of his weakened immune system. His diabetes consultant and GP told him to look after himself properly when he was ill, but he didn't know what that meant, other than that he should rest. When Michael felt another cold coming on, he bought a carton of orange juice and drank it in the belief he was doing himself good. Two days later he was admitted to hospital with a BG level of 25.2 mmol/L and a high level of ketones in his urine. Michael was put on an insulin drip and was told that he should have monitored his BG levels every two or three

2   Jarvis, S. & Rubin, A. (2003), *Diabetes for Dummies*. (Chichester: John Wiley & Sons, Ltd.), p.59.

hours; increased his insulin by one third to cover the extra glucose produced during an infection; and that the high amount of fruit sugar in the orange juice he was drinking had increased his BG and caused his ketoacidosis to be more serious.

FACT: *Diabulimia* – deliberately under-dosing on insulin to lose weight – occurs in 1 in every 400 males and 1 in every 50 females; equal to one-third of all adults taking insulin. This means additional admissions to hospital with diabetic ketoacidosis for these people as they are not taking enough insulin.

Treatment of DKA

DKA is classed as a medical emergency. If you have to be admitted to hospital with DKA, you should understand the treatment you will receive so you know what to expect. Because there is a chemical imbalance in your body, your system will be acidic and lacking water as high BG levels cause the excretion of more urine to flush out glucose and ketone by-products from the breakdown of fat and protein. Health professionals aim to provide treatment to reduce the acidity level of your blood, replace the level of potassium that is lost, and to stabilise BG back down to normal levels.

Each of these levels will be regularly measured by hospital staff and charted so a record can be kept of improvements. You will be put onto an intravenous drip to give a large quantity of vital fluids, potassium, insulin and other necessary medications. Because the body responds very well to the insulin that it needs so badly, BG levels stabilise quickly and may even reach hypo levels. Hospital staff will detect this with regular BG tests and the insulin in the drip may be replaced by a glucose/insulin solution. Once BG goes back down to stable levels, your body will begin to work normally again, ceasing to use fat and protein for fuel. Ketones in the blood from the breakdown of fat and protein will be excreted from the body.

As your body recovers and chemical balance is restored, you will stop feeling and being sick and your brain will be able to function properly. You will be encouraged to take sips of water to make sure your stomach can tolerate it and, as long as you are not sick, you will be allowed to drink water and eat solid food. When the doctor caring for you feels you have recovered, your intravenous drip will be removed and you'll be able to start injecting insulin again.

Low blood glucose – hypoglycaemia

HYPOGLYCAEMIA is the medical term for low blood glucose. If you have diabetes, having a hypo is something you will experience from time to time. Low BG levels of 4.0 mmol/L or less can be owing to an excess of insulin or BG-lowering medication and not enough available glucose. Hypoglycaemia can happen because of the timing of your insulin injections or medication – the food you eat may not be digested at the same time as the insulin or medication is working. You may then have a high BG later on once the food is digested because there's not enough insulin or BG-lowering medication available or it's already stopped working. If you are having hypos before meals and high BG readings later on, this is probably what's happening.

> FACT: Always treat hypoglycaemia as soon as possible with glucose tablets so that the glucose is quickly absorbed into your blood stream to raise levels. Eating something sweet if you don't have glucose tablets may take longer to work as your body has to break down the food to be able to use the glucose.

FACT: If you tend to have severe hypos where your BG drops very low and you pass out, you need to have a Glucagen injection kit in the house and for another person to know where it is and how to use it. If you don't recover, or have a second hypo after Glucagen is given, an ambulance is needed so they can give you intravenous glucose.

You can't always stop a hypo from happening, but you can control it by taking action quickly. You should speak to your diabetes nurse or consultant so they can advise you about how to make the correct adjustments in the timing of your medication dosages. Here's a few other reasons why your BG might drop:

Medication

If you've changed the dosage of insulin or BG-lowering medication, you may have more hypos. The timing of your injections or tablets may also be the reason, as insulin is possibly doing its job of lowering BG when there's less food for it to work on. Remember that different types of insulin work at different times, so make sure you know when yours has its peak working time – the time you are most likely to have a hypo if there's not enough food available. If you miss a meal or take your insulin too early, your BG level will become low. If you take sulphonylurea medication for Type 2 diabetes and you are eating less, your medication will need to be reduced. If you take *sulphonylureas* or a combination of diabetes medication that includes sulphonylureas, these can cause hypoglycaemia. Eat a snack mid-morning and mid-afternoon to avoid low BG at these times and tell your diabetes nurse or GP Practice Nurse about this.

EXERCISE

If you take **moderate exercise** for 20–45 minutes three times a week that **doesn't** get you out of breath this is good for your heart; moderate exercise for 20–30 minutes a day can help you to control your BG levels after meals. When you exercise in a moderate, paced way it generally burns BG and this means you may become hypo. If you plan to take **moderate** exercise, you should lower your insulin or increase your carbohydrate intake so that you don't become low during or afterwards. It is also possible to use exercise to manage your BG levels and avoid taking extra insulin if, for example, your BG is slightly raised to 10 mmol/L when you want it to be 6.5 mmol/L.

FACT: Moderate exercise means different things to different people. If you haven't exercised regularly, cycling very slowly on an exercise bike might be moderate; for a regular exerciser it might be low. Remember, it's moderate if it *doesn't* get you out of breath.

- Build up your exercise endurance to steadily improve your cardiovascular health.
- Muscles, ligaments and tendons become shorter over time with diabetes. Do exercises regularly that strengthen your muscles and build up muscular endurance so that your body benefits from the effort and you feel fitter and healthier.
- Aim to increase how flexible you are by setting goals – for example, aiming to be able to touch your toes with your legs straight, if you can't already.
- If you are overweight, choose exercises that burn body fat – such as swimming, cycling or using a treadmill.

The good news is, the more you weigh, the more calories you burn off just for your body to function every day, and even more if you're physically active. If you are exercising to lose weight as well as trying to reduce BG levels, the following table[3]

3   www.health.harvard.edu/heart

shows calories burned off by doing different activities for ten minutes according to how much you weigh in pounds (lbs):

Activity per 10 minutes	125 lbs	150lbs	175lbs	200lbs
Climbing stairs	150	175	202	229
Running at a pace of a mile in 9 minutes	109	131	153	174
Aerobics – high intensity	95	115	134	153
Swimming – moderate pace	78	90	103	116
Tennis	75	90	105	120
Weight training	66	76	87	98
Cycling at a speed of 10 miles per hour	55	64	78	82
Golf – pulling a golf cart/ carrying clubs	46	54	62	70
Hiking	45	52	60	67
Walking at a pace of a mile in 15 minutes	44	52	61	70
Gardening	41	49	57	65
Shopping	35	42	49	56
Standing	20	24	28	32
Bowling	12	14	16	19
Sitting – reading or watching TV	10	12	14	16
Sleeping	10	12	14	16

FACT: Having an active lifestyle reduces your risk of developing Type 2 diabetes but you may still develop insulin-resistance syndrome – a group of associated conditions including coronary heart disease; high blood pressure; high levels of blood fats such as cholesterol; high levels of chemicals that prevent the breakdown of blood clots in the arteries and heart; and obesity.

Case study: Karen

Karen Mann had been enjoying a daily morning run for three months and, by doing this, managed to reduce her insulin needs by burning off excess blood glucose. Before she started this routine, Karen's morning BG was often around 8.5 mmol/L with an HbA1c of 7.5 per cent (58 mmol/L). Karen made sure she tested her BG before her run and ate a banana to boost her carbohydrate intake to avoid hypos. Her HbA1c now averages around 6.0 per cent (42 mmol/L).

Although exercise burns glucose, your BG can actually **increase** after exercise. This is because:

- Adrenaline released by the liver when you exercise increases BG levels, but if you have some insulin working, this available glucose will be used during the exercise.
- You have eaten too much carbohydrate to avoid a hypo because you thought it would be burned off during exercise. You may not need extra food if your BG levels are high – above 10 mmol/L but less than 16.6 mmol/L – or if you exercise for 20 minutes or less.
- Your BG control is generally not good and there is not enough available insulin working when you exercise. This high BG can cause dangerous ketones – fat and protein being used as fuel instead of glucose – so check your BG is stable before exercising. If you do test positive for ketones with high BG levels and have insulin prescribed to you, take some – 1 unit of insulin usually reduces BG by 1.5 mmol/L, but ask your consultant or diabetes nurse for guidance. **Do not exercise** if your BG is 16.6 mmol/L or above as your heart then has to work much harder to pump syrup-like blood.

FACT: Intense exercise can cause the liver to release stored glucose, increasing BG levels rather than lowering them. This is because when we take intense exercise, there is a seven- to eightfold increase in glucose production in the body and the muscles use only half of it.

As you've just seen under the section about *hyperglycaemia*, if the exercise you do is intense, there must be some insulin working to deal with the stored glucose released by your liver to fuel the muscles.

FACT: Eat complex carbohydrates like bread, potatoes, pasta or rice twenty minutes before you start exercising and keep a sugary drink with you to avoid hypos while exercising.

Research shows that a lack of physical activity is closely associated with a poor quality of life. This means that you can take control and increase the amount of activity you do straight away; do it regularly and make it a lifestyle change to improve your diabetes.

FACT: It's easier to make a change in your lifestyle after receiving information that relates to you and your health personally, such as being told that you have an increased risk of developing Type 2 diabetes.

ALCOHOL

Alcohol acts in several ways to reduce your BG, but then later raises it again when it's been processed by the body. This is because alcohol[4]:

- Stops your liver from releasing glucose.
- Blocks other hormones that raise BG when it's low.
- Increases the BG-lowering effect of insulin so that it works more rapidly.

You might not think of alcohol as a cause of low BG, especially if you have a drink and haven't noticed any problems. These three effects on BG mean that drinking alcohol can cause hypoglycaemia. This is more likely to happen if you are dieting or you don't eat very much generally, especially if you drink alcohol before bed and have a hypo the following morning. This is called *fasting hypoglycaemia*.

Certain drinks, such as vodka and gin, will lower BG so you are more likely to have a hypo. Drinking vodka and orange juice on the other hand will increase BG because of the fruit sugar in the juice. When you have diabetes, it is more important than ever that you drink alcohol only in moderation.

> **FACT: If you take insulin or sulphonylurea medication, always eat some carbohydrate if you're drinking alcohol as this helps stop BG falling too low.**

Different alcoholic drinks contain differing amounts of carbohydrate, so always check the label to be sure. There is a substantial difference between the carbohydrate content of regular and light beer, for example, with regular beer containing 12.8g per 370ml bottle, while the same amount of light beer provides only 5.8g of carbohydrate. White wine also varies among brands and

---

4   Jarvis, S. & Rubin, A. (2003), *Diabetes for Dummies* (Chichester: John Wiley & Sons Ltd.) p.57.

grape varieties, but is typically 2.8g of carbohydrate for a 125ml serving of Chardonnay over the same amount of Riesling at 4.5g of carbs.

ASPIRIN

Aspirin, particularly in large doses, can lower BG. This is especially the case for people with Type 2 diabetes who take BG-lowering medication containing sulphonylureas[5], as aspirin helps the tablets do their job more effectively. Doctors thought at one time that this combination could be used as a different form of treatment for Type 2, but the effects on BG weren't always the same, so they abandoned the idea. The Department of Health has advised that every adult with diabetes should take a small 75mg dose of aspirin daily to protect against the risk of stroke and heart disease. Some over-the-counter aspirin tablets contain four times this amount – 300mg – and if you are used to swallowing two aspirin if you have a headache, this is not only a high dosage, but it can also significantly lower your BG. This is because aspirin can also increase the way other BG-lowering drugs work, but I've not found this to be the case with insulin.

FACT: Children should never take aspirin.

Mild hypos make you feel uncomfortable, but they're **not** dangerous. If you ignore how you're feeling and don't test your blood and eat something sweet to treat the hypo, your BG may drop even lower to become a **severe** hypo. This can be dangerous if you are on your own and lose consciousness, or if other people don't know what action to take. Always test your BG if you feel unwell because some symptoms of low and high BG are similar and everyone with diabetes experiences different warning signs. Common signs of hypo are:

5   Jarvis, S. & Rubin, A. (2003), *Diabetes for Dummies* (Chichester: John Wiley & Sons Ltd.), p.261.

Mild Signs

- Sweating
- Hunger
- Rapid heartbeat

Moderate Signs

- Irritable/aggressive behaviour
- Muscle weakness

For both mild or moderate hypos, test your BG and if you are low, eat something sweet: 2–4 glucose tablets; a glass of pure orange juice or Lucozade; a small glass of non-diet fizzy drink. Follow this up with carbohydrate such as a couple of digestive biscuits, a slice of bread, or a banana. Wait for 15–20 minutes and test again. If you are still low, get something else to eat or a cup of tea with sugar. If you are very disorientated, this should be done by a **hypo partner**.

Severe Signs

- Blurred vision
- Drowsiness
- Clumsiness/appearing to be drunk
- Confusion
- Passing out – unconsciousness
- Losing the ability to shiver if you're cold

If you have a severe hypo and can't swallow – remember, it's dangerous to feed an unconscious person in case they choke – *Hypostop* is a sugary gel that can be smeared on the lips or gums so it's absorbed into the bloodstream quickly. If you become unconscious, you will need another person to take **emergency action** by mixing and injecting glucagen from a hypo kit. You will also need to have a sugary drink when you regain consciousness. If you don't become conscious, someone should dial 999.

NIGHT-TIME HYPOS

Many people who take insulin to treat their diabetes fear night-time hypos – *nocturnal hypoglycaemia* – when they are asleep and not able to monitor their BG or detect hypo symptoms as they would when they're awake. Some also fear that they might have a hypo in their sleep and not wake up. This can also be a big worry for your partner and your family, and for parents of children with Type 1 diabetes. While there is more likelihood that a hypo won't be detected as quickly during sleep, your brain will let you know that it needs glucose:

- You'll be woken up with symptoms of feeling shaky and sweaty, restless and irritable.
- If applicable, restlessness in bed will disturb your partner's sleep and they will wake you up so you can treat your hypo with glucose.
- Even if your hypo is severe, your body has a mechanism to release stored glucose from the liver when BG levels fall, and this happens even when you remain asleep.

You'll wake up with a bad headache and feel generally unwell, similar to a hangover. Because of this BG 'auto-correction' in response to hypo, high BG levels follow. Regularly waking and feeling like this, and finding that your BG is high, may indicate that your BG is falling very low in your sleep. Occasionally test your BG at 3 a.m. to make sure this isn't happening. If your levels are dipping in the night, speak to your diabetes consultant or diabetes nurse for advice on altering your insulin dosages or diet to prevent it happening again.

FACT: If you become unconscious, you may clench your teeth because of low BG. It is also important that your hypo partner doesn't try to feed you anything to eat or drink when you're unconscious as you may choke.

Hypoglycaemic unawareness

Sometimes there are no symptoms of hypo. This can happen when you've had diabetes for many years and is associated with nerve damage. It can also happen if you have to take heart or blood pressure medication, where your hypo symptoms will be less obvious to you. The danger of hypoglycaemic unawareness is that you may not recognise a hypo during your sleep, so you fail to wake up from it and fall into unconsciousness. Another danger is to have a hypo without warning while driving. In such circumstances, you have an increased need to test your BG frequently throughout the day and during the night to detect low BG results.

I have hypo unawareness owing to long-duration diabetes. It caused me problems until I began using a Continuous Glucose Monitoring – *CGM* – system with my insulin pump ten years ago. CGM is a sensor inserted under the skin and changed every six days to provide continual updates on BG levels every ten minutes via an insulin-pump display screen. The insulin pump sounds an alarm if my BG levels fall below 4.0 mmol/L. In this way, I'm able to take action when the pump notifies me that my BG is dropping down low, and I can avoid becoming unconscious during a severe hypo.

> FACT: If you have frequent and unpredictable hypoglycaemia with no warning signs, you're a good candidate for NHS-funded insulin-pump therapy and CGM. Speak to your diabetes consultant or GP to find out more.

Flash sensor bg testing

New technology now means that BG can be tested without a finger-prick blood sample. The scanning *flash glucose sensor* is a device the size of a £2 coin that uses a probe inserted just under the skin on the back of the arm to measure plasma glucose by reading a signal. This device for people with

Type 1 diabetes has been available on the NHS since November 2017, but some people have found that it is still not funded in their area of the UK. One disadvantage of the device is that BG can be self-checked only when the person is awake – although a parent can check their child's BG during the night. While the measurement of plasma glucose is not as accurate as the measurement of BG, this device allows better management of Type 1 diabetes.

THE EFFECTS OF SEVERE HYPOGLYCAEMIA

Having a severe hypo makes you feel very disorientated as your brain adjusts to having suffered low BG levels and a lack of glucose for fuel. Because of this it is a very good idea to have someone you trust who can help you during these situations. Everyone has different experiences of what it's like to have extremely low BG, and people who know you well can see that you are not behaving normally, so will take action. During the hypo it's practically impossible to explain to others what it feels like because your glucose-starved brain is in a state of confusion.

You may never experience the effects of severe hypoglycaemia – meaning a BG of less than 2.0 mmol/L (36 mg/dl in the USA), where *Glucagen* has to be injected by another person because you're unconscious, but if you do, I've tried to describe below how it feels:

- After initial sweating and feeling very hot, severe low BG levels lead to a dramatic drop in body temperature – *hypothermia* – and an inability to get warm.
- Muscle weakness and confusion last for several hours after coming out of unconsciousness because the brain and body are deprived of glucose for fuel.
- A severe headache lasts for the rest of the day, and sometimes the following day as well.
- Because the body needs to replace stores of glucose in the liver, there is an extreme feeling of hunger and a compulsion to eat a large amount of food. Inevitably this, coupled with the release of glucose

from the liver to correct hypoglycaemia, results in a very high BG hours later. This leads to feeling very sick.

- While unconscious, some – like myself – experience epileptic-like fits because the brain has been starved of glucose and this causes some brain cells to die off. Because of this, after recovery, I had a complete loss of memory of events immediately before the severe hypo.

FACT: As long as you have warning signs and act quickly, treat your hypo as soon as you realise it's happening so you won't become unconscious or need the help of other people.

HOW OFTEN SHOULD I TEST MY BG?

When you are first diagnosed with diabetes, you will be asked to test your BG more frequently than when it's stabilised. If you have Type 1 diabetes or you have Type 2 and you take insulin, it's advisable to test BG before meals, before driving and before bed. This is because you can make insulin adjustments according to each meal. So, if you have a BG of 13 mmol/L and normally have a set dose of insulin for your evening meal, you can take a correction dosage of a couple more units to deal with the glucose you already have in your blood, as well as the meal you will eat. On some evenings, you may eat a more or less carbohydrate-rich meal, so the insulin you take could be too little or too much to keep BG in check.

FACT: One great way to take control of your diabetes is to write the carbohydrate values of your favourite foods in a notebook, so you can quickly calculate your insulin needs.

There are people with diabetes who have frequent and unpredictable hypos with little or no warning. If this is relevant to you, you need to carry out more BG tests to give you the confidence to be independent and in control of your condition. If you forget to test your blood occasionally throughout the day or night, it's not something to worry about. By getting into a regular routine, you will be on the right track for keeping your BG under control.

Case study: Paul

Paul Maxwell was prescribed a BG-lowering medication that had a peak working time of two to four hours after taking it. Because Paul ate his evening meal at 8 p.m. and then went to bed a couple of hours later, he found he was having hypos during the night. Paul had been advised that he needed to test his BG only three times a week because he had Type 2 diabetes, but he began to test before bed every night. He found that his BG was often only 4.0–4.5 mmol/L and reported this to his GP. With some adjustments to his evening carbohydrate count and his sulphonylurea dosage, Paul was able to retire to bed without the worry of having night-time hypos.

FACT: You should always test your BG before you go to sleep.

If you try to tighten your BG control, for example, if you are pregnant and keeping your diabetes as well controlled as possible for the developing baby, you may have more hypos because there is less available glucose before you go too low. If you do make changes by increasing your insulin and you feel unwell, it is important to test BG to make sure you're not having a hypo.

Case study: Me!

The body's reaction to low BG changes over the years. Now I've had Type 1 diabetes for 41 years, I find that I don't always feel the same when I have low BG. Sometimes I feel really tired and hot during the day or I get a bad headache – symptoms I've realised may be owing to low BG rather than just normal life. I always test in case it's a hypo, despite what the glucose sensor tells me, so I can then take action to raise BG levels if I need to.

If you have Type 2 diabetes that's treated by tablets, diet and exercise, you may be advised to check your BG levels before breakfast and dinner, but if your HbA1c level is in the 'good' range, you may need to test only two to three times a week. If you take sulphonylurea medication, which can cause hypoglycaemia, you should test your BG several times a day. In the USA and in some other countries, the thinking is that frequent testing for people with Type 2 diabetes does very little to improve BG control, especially as taking tablets allows no flexibility in controlling BG in the same way taking insulin does. This is because, without being able to take additional insulin when you have a high BG level, there is little you can do to lower it, other than to exercise.

> **FACT: Always wash your hands before testing your BG as it can make a big difference to the result.**

Doing repeated BG tests, especially if your consultant is trying to stabilise your insulin treatment, can make your fingers very sore. The good news is that there are alternatives for getting a blood sample other than the fingertips, allowing your fingers to have a rest. The bad news is that getting blood from sites like the upper arm, forearm, thigh or lower leg may not give an accurate reading, because the glucose level in these parts of the body is 20–30 minutes older than in the fingertips. The fingertips and palm provide the most up-to-date BG readings. Because of this lag, avoid using alternative sites for blood testing if:

- You don't get many or any hypo warning signs – *hypoglycaemic unawareness.*
- You are feeling low and need to know **how** low.
- You are ill and your BG levels are running higher from infection.
- You are just about to drive a vehicle.

Case study: Kim

Kim Davies was 22 and had just been diagnosed with Type 1 diabetes. She was having difficulty getting her insulin dosages stable and her diabetes nurse advised that she should test her BG eight to ten times a day. Her fingertips were taking a battering, but she persevered because she knew this would not be a long-term situation and because her BG tended to drop very quickly. After three weeks, Kim was able to monitor her BG using alternative sites and reduce the number of tests to four per day.

Chapter 6

LIFESTYLE CHANGE

'I realised that my Type 2 diabetes was completely a result of lifestyle factors.'

The key message concerning many cases of Type 2 diabetes is that you *can* do something about it. I will be covering reversing Type 2 diabetes later, but it is possible to improve your BG levels enormously just by making a few small changes. Making small lifestyle changes can be hugely beneficial if you have either Type 1 or Type 2 diabetes.

FACT: One in ten adults now risk developing Type 2 diabetes by the year 2035.

Case Study: Chris

Chris Jenkins was 54 and weighed 127kg when he was told he had Type 2 diabetes. He told his doctor that eating and drinking were his only pleasures and because he enjoyed food, he wondered what was the point of making lifestyle changes to include diet and exercise. Chris saw his diabetes consultant for the first time and he agreed that Chris's diabetes was completely lifestyle-related. He added that Chris could improve his condition markedly if he steadily lost weight and did regular fat-burning exercise like cycling. Chris's family wanted him to be well and they encouraged him to follow this advice. He cut out cake, biscuits, chips and crisps from his diet and took up cycling for 8km three times a week with his daughter. At Chris's next clinic appointment, he was happy to be told his diabetes was now borderline and that he could actually say goodbye to his Type 2 if he made his lifestyle changes permanent. Chris felt so much better that he did exactly that. He no longer takes Metformin.

FACT: Health problems related to poor diet, drinking and smoking are currently costing the NHS £11 billion each year.

STARCHES AND SUGARS

As you have seen in the last chapter, eating any sort of carbohydrate will increase your BG, but there are different forms of carbohydrate. Potatoes, pasta and bread contain starch – good carbohydrates. Sweets, cakes and biscuits are bad carbohydrates that will raise your BG quickly and provide little nutritional value because they contain glucose or sugar. Modern diets now contain far too many bad carbohydrates and this, along with a sedentary lifestyle with little or no exercise, is the reason for the sharp rise in obesity and associated Type 2 diabetes in recent years. By monitoring your BG regularly, you will be able to see exactly how eating good and bad carbohydrates causes BG-level fluctuations.

It's not always easy to know which foods contain sugars that will adversely affect your BG levels – foods such as tomato sauce and pickled onions are culprits that I find often catch people out. Furthermore, low-fat foods, which we might think are healthy, can fool us into thinking we're making good choices, but manufacturers often increase the amount of sugar in low-fat foods in order to replace lost flavour.

Always **read food labels** to check exactly – if glucose syrup or sugar is the first thing on the ingredients list, you can be sure that particular food is not for you. I once bought cranberry juice that didn't taste particularly sweet, but my BG shot up to somewhere in the twenties after a small glass. I tested a drop of cranberry juice on a BG-monitoring stick (which is not designed for this purpose, but it worked). The reading said 'HI'. It wasn't just being friendly – this meant the reading was so high, the meter couldn't read the glucose content. The cranberry drink was packed with sugar; like drinking flavoured glucose in juice form. I now always buy unsweetened juice, which still has natural sugar in it, but no added sugar at all.

FACT: **If foods are marked 'low sugar', it means they contain no more than 5 per cent sugar per 100g/100ml of food or drink. Foods marked 'high sugar' have 15g sugar per 100g/100ml, so avoid these for the sake of your BG.**

CARBOHYDRATES

Being aware of how much carbohydrate there is in certain foods can help you match your diabetes medication and exercise to the food you eat. The trouble is that some carbohydrates raise BG more than others – **all carbohydrates are not the same.** You may have heard of *glycaemic index* – GI – diets based on foods that raise BG the least. This is decided by how quickly your body absorbs the carbohydrate in food to convert it to glucose for fuel. The good news is that by making a few simple substitutions in your diet, you can start eating low-GI foods that raise your BG much less than high-GI foods, helping you have a stable BG with fewer ups and downs.

But sometimes, it's not that simple because[1]:

- The GI of some foods may be different when eaten alone compared with if they're eaten as part of a meal.
- If you are eating, for example, a cheese sandwich, the protein and fat in the cheese can increase the GI value of the meal.
- Foods that are processed may have a different GI value to the unprocessed versions of the same foods.
- Although chocolate is a low GI food because it takes time to increase your BG, it has a lot of calories from fat, so it can't help you lose weight.

FACT: Don't eat chocolate to treat a hypo as it takes a long time to raise BG levels.

For these reasons, the low-GI diet hasn't become part of general diabetes management because it can be complicated. There are books you can buy on this subject that list the GI value of every food so you can make choices to suit you. A few changes you can make in your diet that will make a big difference to your glucose levels are[2]:

- Swap white or wholemeal bread – high-GI foods – for wholegrain bread, which contains slow-release carbohydrate.
- Eat porridge oats instead of other corn- or wheat-based cereals – oats raise your BG slowly and also reduce cholesterol.
- Include biscuits/bars that contain dried fruits or grains in your diet.
- Swap high-fat, high-sugar cakes for healthy options made with whole

1   Jarvis, S. & Rubin, A. (2003), *Diabetes for Dummies* (Chichester: John Wiley & Sons Ltd.), p.139.
2   Ibid., p.139.

grains and fruits – this means something like a Nutrigrain bar, not an apple turnover!

- Choose fruit that is raw or under-ripe as this contains less fruit sugar than over-ripe fruit.
- Eat a piece of fruit – not bananas, pineapple, mango, guava or passion fruit, which contain a lot of carbohydrate – rather than drinking a glass of fruit juice.
- Swap older potatoes and instant mash for boiled new potatoes – the older the potato, the more carbohydrate it contains.
- Eat rice or pasta instead of potatoes. Long-grain rice has more carbohydrate than Basmati rice, so read the labels and compare values before buying.
- Choose peas or beans – not baked beans in a tin with tomato sauce – as they are full of slow-release carbohydrates.

Because lower GI foods can make such a difference to your BG control, you will need to check your BG more often if you decide to start a low-GI diet to reduce your glucose levels. Make sure you tell your diabetes nurse or your GP Practice Nurse before you begin as they can help you manage your diabetes while you are making these changes. There is a lot of information to take in and consider with a low-GI diet, so you may decide it's not for you. Your diabetes diet, on the other hand, needs to have a certain amount of carbohydrate – low GI or not – for your insulin or BG medication to work.

The carbohydrate content of common foods is shown below[3]:

Food	Carbohydrate
1 cup of cooked white pasta or rice	45g
1 English muffin	30g
1 medium potato	30g
1 cup of sweetcorn or peas	30g
Half a cup of cooked vegetables – carrots/broccoli/green beans	15g

3   'Getting to Grips with Type 2 Diabetes' (2010). See www.desmond-project.co.uk.

1 slice of bread	15g
1 small piece of fruit – apple/satsuma/nectarine	15g
17 grapes or 12 cherries	15g
Half a cup of vanilla ice cream	15g
2 small, plain biscuits	15g
1 cup of milk	12g

FACT: In a diabetic diet, one serving of carbohydrate is measured as 15 grams.

Different foods with the same amount of carbohydrate raise BG in the same way, so a serving of two medium potatoes has the same carbohydrate content as four slices of bread – 60g.

FACT: It is the *amount* of carbohydrate that is important, not the *type*.

You may think that choosing a sugar-free version of a food is better for you, but beware – low-sugar foods can still be **high in carbohydrates**. For example, a sugar-free yoghurt is not made with sugar, but the natural sugar – lactose – in the milk that makes the yoghurt means it will increase your BG if you eat it.

When your diabetes is first diagnosed you may be advised to eat a certain amount of carbohydrate every day to balance your diabetes medication. You don't have to eat the same thing at each meal every day. As long as the carbohydrate value is the same as you've been advised, you can have the meal of your choice. It can be very easy to eat more than you planned because of portion sizes.

> TIP: Always read food labels so you can see exactly the amount
> of carbohydrate, fat and calories you are eating.

The NHS advises that, depending on whether you are male or female, you need a certain amount of carbohydrate every day[4]. Women need 30–60g of carbohydrate for their main meals and 15–30g for snacks. Men need 45–75g of carbohydrate for their main meals and 15–30g for snacks. Weight-loss diets will contain reduced carbohydrate portions and you will be advised how to make these changes by your GP and/or diabetes team. To prevent low and high swings in BG:

- Don't miss meals.
- Space your meals regularly throughout the day.
- Eat balanced meals of carbohydrate, lean protein and healthy fat.

GOOD FATS AND BAD FATS

Case study: Julie

Julie Morris was 40, had Type 2 diabetes and ate a high-fat diet. She found losing weight very difficult and her BG levels were usually high when she tested them. Julie's doctor warned her that heart disease is very common in people with Type 2 diabetes, but she said her parents and grandparents had always eaten fatty meat, butter, cheese and cream so she did the same without realising that these foods had an effect on her BG levels.

4   'Getting to Grips with Type 2 Diabetes' (2010). See www.desmond-project.co.uk.

There are many types of fat. Some, like olive oil, are good for the body while others are bad, increasing *insulin resistance* – meaning that insulin cannot work properly – and levels of cholesterol (blood fats). All fats contain many calories and eating them regularly can mean it's hard to lose weight. The table below[5] shows the different types of good and bad fat:

Good fats – monounsaturated	Medium fats – polyunsaturated	Bad fats – saturated fats
Rapeseed oil Olive oil – including butter substitutes	Sunflower oil Corn oil Soya oil Low-fat spreads – labelled high in polyunsaturates	Butter Lard Block cooking fats Ghee butter and solid oils Hard margarine Fats found in pies, pastry, sausages, cakes, biscuits and full-fat cheeses

> **FACT:** Where fat is concerned, if you generally eat low-fat, low-sugar foods your BG levels will be better controlled than if you often eat many high-fat foods – such as pies, cakes, crisps, chips and biscuits.

As well as checking food labels for sugar and glucose, it is also wise to check the fat content before you buy. This does depend on how often you eat the food and, of course, how much you eat – eating the occasional plate of cheese and biscuits is not the same as a daily sausage roll or slice of cake.

- Foods that are labelled low in fat must contain less than 3g of fat per 100g or 100ml.

5   'Getting to Grips with Type 2 Diabetes' (2010). See www.desmond-project.co.uk.

- Reduced-fat foods must contain 25 per cent less fat than a full-fat version – but if it's something like a butter substitute, it is still generally high in fat. This also goes for any light version of a full-fat product.

FACT: Insulin helps the body to lay down fat stores by converting glucose and other nutrients into fatty acids.

Fruit and veg

The NHS encourages us to eat at least five portions of fruit and vegetables a day as a source of valuable vitamins and minerals. People with diabetes are often short of B vitamins, necessary for a healthy nervous system; zinc, needed for growth; and vitamin D to help maintain – amongst other things – a healthy immune system. (Vitamin D may be short if you don't go outside much because you are working, disabled or elderly, so check with your doctor, especially if you frequently feel tired.) So, what counts as a 'portion'?

ONE portion of our five a day is[6]:

- One apple or orange, or other medium fruit.
- Two smaller fruits, such as plums or satsumas.
- Three tablespoons of tinned fruit in natural fruit juice (DON'T eat fruit in syrup).
- One dessert-sized bowl of salad.
- Two tomatoes.
- Three tablespoons of cooked vegetables.

6 'Getting to Grips with Type 2 Diabetes' (2010). See www.desmond-project.co.uk.

> **FACT:** Avoid buying fruit or vegetables that are unwrapped, don't need peeling, and are exposed to traffic fumes, as they can contain toxic heavy metals such as lead, aluminium, cadmium, mercury and arsenic from pollution.

VITAMINS

Where can we find our vitamins and what do they do in the body?

- Vitamin A is found in liver, milk, carrots and green vegetables and it is needed for healthy bones and skin.
- Vitamin B1 – also known as *thiamine* – is found in meat and wholegrain cereals and is necessary for the body to convert carbohydrates into energy.
- Vitamin B2 – also known as *riboflavin* – is found in milk, cheese, fish and green vegetables and is needed for the correct metabolism of food.
- Vitamin B3 – also known as *niacin* – is found in fish, lean meat, and nuts and is essential for the release of energy in the body. It is also necessary for memory and healthy cardiovascular function.
- Vitamin B5 – also known as *pantothenic acid* – is found in avocados, broccoli, meat, porridge, tomatoes and whole grains and is needed to break down protein, fats and carbohydrate for energy and for re-building tissues, muscles and organs.
- Vitamin B6 – also known as *pyridoxine* – can be found in liver, yeast, Marmite and brown bread. It is essential for growth.
- Vitamin B12 is found in meat and Marmite and is needed for a healthy nervous system and red blood cells.
- *Folic acid* – also known as Vitamin B9 – is found in green leafy vegetables, potatoes, wholegrain bread, and breakfast cereals with added vitamins. The body needs it for the general maintenance of a healthy nervous system and red blood cells and is essential during pregnancy.

- Vitamin C is found in fruit and potatoes and is needed for the maintenance of body tissues.
- Vitamin D is found in milk, cheese and yoghurt. The body also manufacturers it from exposure to sunlight. Along with calcium, it is necessary for strong bones and teeth.
- Vitamin E is found in wheat germ, wholegrain cereals, and vegetable oils and is needed for the maintenance of body cells.
- Vitamin K is produced by the bacteria that live in your intestines and can also be found in leafy green vegetables. It is essential for blood clotting and wound healing.

FACT: If you have Type 2 diabetes and have been prescribed *Orlistat* – also known as Xenical – to manage obesity, you may be deficient in fat-soluble vitamins as a result. Orlistat works by stopping around a third of the fat you eat from being digested, so this reduces absorption of some fat-soluble vitamin supplements, particularly vitamins A and E. Orlistat should not be taken with Acarbose diabetes medication.

We need some vitamins on a daily basis because they are water-soluble and are washed out of the body in the urine. These vitamins include all the B vitamins and vitamin C. Vitamins A, D, E and K are stored in fat globules in the bloodstream, small intestine and body tissues so we rarely run out. In fact, we may have too much of them, resulting in a condition called *hyper-vitaminosis*, which can be harmful and is caused by taking an excess of vitamin supplements.

People with both Type 1 diabetes and coeliac disease – an intolerance to gluten – can have a vitamin-D deficiency and you may need to take pre-scribed, rather than over-the-counter supplements. Always seek advice from your doctor or dietician about taking vitamin and mineral supplements as you may need specific amounts.

MINERALS

Where can we find our vitamins and what do they do in the body?

The body needs some minerals, such as calcium, as 'building blocks' for repair and renewal. It needs others, like sodium and potassium, for correct nerve and muscle function. These minerals are known as *electrolytes*. Ketoacidosis associated with high BG levels upsets the balance of minerals in the body, as the body becomes more acidic. In severe cases, ketoacidosis is a medical emergency needing hospitalisation to have the body's chemical balance restored. The main role minerals have in the body is to help enzymes turn one substance into another, such as the breakdown of proteins to make new body cells.

> **FACT:** **All minerals are toxic to the body in large amounts. Some minerals, like chromium, have different forms and one variety may be toxic while another is essential to us. Some minerals reduce the action of other minerals in the body – for example, iron can cause zinc deficiency because it blocks zinc from working.**

- Calcium, phosphorus and magnesium can be found in milk, yoghurt and cheese. We need these for strong bones and teeth. Adults should get 1,000mg per day[7]. Growing teenagers, pregnant women and older people need 1,500mg every day. Calcium and vitamin D work together in the body.

---

7   Holford, P. (1992), *Optimum Nutrition: How to Get the Very Best Out of Yourself* (London: ION Press).

> **FACT:** BG-lowering medication can cause magnesium deficiency, ketoacidosis and irregular heart rhythm (*cardiac arrhythmia*) and you may need to take magnesium supplements.

- Magnesium helps convert food into energy and is important for bone health. It can be found in green leafy vegetables like spinach, nuts, brown rice, bread (especially wholegrain), fish, meat and dairy foods. Magnesium deficiency is quite common.
- Potassium is vital for the healthy function of body cells, tissues and organs and helps control water balance and blood acidity levels in the body. It is found in bananas, avocados, spinach, lentils and all fruits and vegetables.
- Selenium is important for brain function and a healthy immune system. It is also necessary for fertility in men and women. The richest source of selenium is brazil nuts – although these are also high in cholesterol – seafood and organ meats such as liver and kidney.
- Zinc helps achieve a healthy immune system and is important for cell division, to prevent cancer, to maintain healthy hormone levels **especially** insulin sensitivity, and good energy levels. Zinc is found in walnuts, Marmite, oysters, wheat germ, beef and veal. However, zinc stops iron, manganese and copper from being absorbed by the body.
- Manganese can be found in many fruits and vegetables, such as bananas, raspberries, strawberries, pineapple, grapes, garlic, green beans, and in rice, nuts and oats. It is needed to maintain a healthy bone structure and brain and nervous system function, and for creating essential enzymes for building bones.
- Iron can be found in meat, dark green leafy vegetables (such as spinach), wholemeal bread, nuts and beans and is needed for the formation of red blood cells. Iron helps form haemoglobin that carries oxygen in the blood: two-thirds of the iron in the body makes up our

haemoglobin. Women who are menstruating and people with certain health conditions can become iron deficient and anaemic, requiring iron supplements. Because iron is stored in the body tissues, a build-up of iron over time can lead to diabetes, arthritis and heart abnormalities.

- Sodium is found in salt and you need only 220mg daily[8]. The body uses sodium to regulate the amount of water it stores. Most people eat far too much sodium in their diet, with elevated blood pressure as a result. Sodium is added to foods such as crisps, breakfast cereals, sauces and processed meats during manufacturing, so don't add additional salt when you're cooking meals from scratch.

- Copper is needed by the body to make red blood cells and to keep nerve cells and the immune system healthy. Deficiency is rare because it is found in drinking water passed through copper pipes. Copper stops zinc and manganese from working.

- Chromium is found in meat, whole grains, fruit, vegetables and spices. Your body needs it only in very small quantities to reduce blood pressure, turn glucose into energy and to help insulin to work. In Type 2 diabetes, 100mg chromium a day is recommended for good BG balance[9].

- Iodine deficiency is extremely rare as this mineral is added to iodised salt. It's necessary for the correct functioning of the thyroid gland in the neck and the production of thyroid hormones, which help the body metabolise food. Iodine is also found in milk, yoghurt, cheese, seafood, mushrooms, meat and eggs.

DEFICIENCY SYMPTOMS

The vitamins you need depend on your general health. Ideally, your intake of vitamins should be a dosage to give you the best possible health with diabetes and to prevent any symptoms of deficiency. This level can be measured only

8 Holford, P. (1992), *Optimum Nutrition: How to Get the Very Best Out of Yourself* (London: ION Press.)
9 Ibid.

by blood tests, but you may need 50–100 times the recommended daily allowance (*RDA*) of some vitamins and minerals.

RDAs vary from country to country, and some essential nutrients don't have an RDA at all. The RDA is the **minimum** amount required for health[10]: it may not be possible to gain everything you need from your diet because of various factors such as how food is grown, where it's stored, how old it is, whether it has been in direct sunlight and how efficient your body is at processing it.

FACT: **Even if we all ate the recommended daily allowance of vitamins and minerals, some people would still have symptoms of deficiencies because we all have different needs.**

It is natural to worry that you could be having too much of a certain vitamin and that it could cause damage because stories in the press highlight these issues. It has been claimed that vitamin A is toxic and harmful during pregnancy; that large doses of vitamin C can cause kidney stones; and that B6 in excess is dangerous for the nervous system.

FACT: **It is unlikely that you would have any symptoms of vitamin overdose from taking a daily multivitamin supplement tablet.**

---

10 Holford, P. (1992), *Optimum Nutrition: How to Get the Very Best Out of Yourself* (London: ION Press).

VITAMIN A comes in an animal form (*retinol*), which is stored in the body, and a vegetable form known as *beta-carotene*, which is found in carrots and converted into retinol by the body if needed. Eating lots of carrots can cause yellowing of the skin because excessive beta-carotene is stored there, but it is not toxic to the body. A variety of synthetic vitamin A supplements – sold as *Roaccutane* – has been shown to cause toxic effects and birth defects because the vitamin A content is very high and the pregnant women involved had taken 25,000–500,000 international units a day.[11]

VITAMIN B6, as with all B-vitamins, is water-soluble and any excess is excreted in the urine. There has been a case of a woman who increased her daily dose of B6 from 50mg to 200mg over a two-year period and she developed some muscle weakness and pain that was diagnosed as nerve damage.[12] Research studies where people took between 2,000mg and 5,000mg of B6 per day showed improvements in nerve function, so it may have been a case that the woman suffering adverse effects had other underlying health problems causing her symptoms.

VITAMIN C is water-soluble and if the body can't use it, any excess is excreted in the urine. There are no associations between vitamin C and kidney stones and the only adverse effect of taking very large dosages – above 3,000mg per day[13] – is that it has a laxative effect.

---

11   Holford, P. (1992), *Optimum Nutrition: How to Get the Very Best Out of Yourself* (London: ION Press).
12   Ibid.
13   Ibid.

> FACT: Supplements contain larger amounts of vitamins that
> are cheaper to produce, like vitamin C. They may
> contain only very small amounts of the vitamins or
> minerals you need, so always ask advice before buying
> them from a healthfood shop.

Deficiency symptoms for each vitamin and mineral[14]:

VITAMIN A
Mouth ulcers; poor night vision; acne; frequent colds or infections; dry, flaky skin; dandruff; diarrhoea; thrush or cystitis.

VITAMIN B1
Tender muscles; eye pains; irritability; poor concentration; 'prickly' legs and tingling hands – also a symptom of diabetic nerve damage; poor memory; stomach pains; rapid heartbeat; constipation (common in people with diabetes).

VITAMIN B2
Burning or gritty eyes; sensitivity to bright light; sore tongue; cataracts (common in people with diabetes owing to high BG over time); dull or oily hair; eczema or dermatitis; split nails; cracked lips.

VITAMIN B3
Lack of energy; insomnia; headaches or migraines; poor memory; anxiety or tension; depression; irritability; bleeding or tender gums; acne.

VITAMIN B5
Muscle tension or cramps; apathy (tiredness/no energy – also a symptom of

14 Holford, P. (1992), *Optimum Nutrition: How to Get the Very Best Out of Yourself* (London: ION Press).

high BG); poor concentration; tender heels; nausea or vomiting; exhaustion after light exercise; anxiety or tension; teeth grinding; burning feet (also a symptom of diabetic neuropathy).

VITAMIN B6
Infrequent dream recall; water retention; tingling hands (also a symptom of peripheral neuropathy); depression and irritability (common in people with diabetes); nervousness; muscle tremors or cramps; lack of energy; flaky skin.

VITAMIN B12
Poor hair condition; eczema or dermatitis; over-sensitivity to hot or cold in the mouth; irritability; anxiety or tension; lack of energy (also a symptom of high BG); constipation (common in people with diabetes); tender, sore muscles; pale skin.

VITAMIN B9 (folic acid)
Eczema; cracked lips; prematurely greying hair; anxiety or tension; poor memory; lack of energy; depression; poor appetite; stomach pains.

VITAMIN C
Frequent colds; lack of energy; frequent infections; bleeding or tender gums; easy bruising; nose bleeds; slow wound healing; red pimples on the skin.

VITAMIN D
Rheumatism or arthritis; backache; tooth decay; hair loss; excessive sweating; muscle cramps or spasms; joint pain or stiffness; lack of energy.

VITAMIN E
Lack of sex drive; exhaustion after light exercise; easy bruising; slow wound healing (common in people with diabetes); varicose veins; loss of muscle tone; infertility.

CALCIUM
Muscle cramps or tremors; insomnia or nervousness; joint pain or arthritis; tooth decay; high blood pressure.

CHROMIUM

Excessive sweating or cold sweats; dizziness or irritability after six hours without food (both a sign of low BG, so make sure you test your blood); cold hands (also a sign of damage to blood vessels in diabetes); need for excessive amounts of sleep or drowsiness during the day; excessive thirst (also a main symptom of diabetes due to high BG levels).

IRON

Pale skin; sore tongue; tiredness/listlessness; loss of appetite or nausea; heavy periods or blood loss.

MAGNESIUM

Muscle tremors or spasms; muscle weakness; insomnia or nervousness; high blood pressure; irregular heartbeat; constipation; fits or convulsions (although not the same as fits that can occur if BG is very low); hyperactivity; depression.

MANGANESE

Muscle twitches; childhood growing pains; dizziness and poor sense of balance (not to be confused with balance problems associated with peripheral nerve damage in diabetes); fits or convulsions; sore knees.

SELENIUM

Family history of cancer; signs of premature ageing – although having diabetes also ages the body's cells more quickly owing to abnormal metabolism; cataracts; high blood pressure; frequent infections.

ZINC

Poor sense of taste or smell; white marks on more than two fingernails; frequent infections; stretch marks; acne or greasy skin; low fertility (also a sign of high BG over time); pale skin; tendency to depression; poor appetite.

CONTROLLING YOUR WEIGHT

By making some changes in the amount of exercise you take and what you eat at every meal, you can really make a difference to your weight. It stands to reason that replacing a chocolate bar with a banana or apple could help you reduce your daily calories. I remember being told this by my sports teacher at school, so it's not a new idea. Basically, a woman needs 2,000 calories a day and a man needs 2,500 so the body can function. If you eat more calories than you need – including those you burn off with exercise, you will put on weight. Calorie counting is an art in itself and, if you want to count everything you eat there are books and Apps available that list the calories in every kind of food you can buy. A quick guide below shows how you can make a difference to your weight and your BG by cutting out a few 100-calorie snacks each day.

Each of these is around 100 calories[15]:

3 chocolate fingers; or 2 custard creams; or 2 Jaffa cakes; or 1½ plain digestive biscuits.

2 tablespoons of double cream; or 30g full-fat cheese; or 15g butter.

1 tablespoon of cooking oil; or 15g sunflower spread.

7 teaspoons of jam; or 6 teaspoons of tomato sauce; or 2 tablespoons of salad cream.

small packet of crisps or 15g salted peanuts.

3 slices of lean turkey; or 2 cocktail sausage rolls; or ½ a mini pork pie.

2 glasses of unsweetened fruit juice; or 1 small glass of white wine; or ½ pint of beer or lager.

As you can see from this list, it's all about making choices. You may eat a couple of biscuits with your coffee or tea, or a packet of crisps without even

---

15 'Getting to Grips with Type 2 Diabetes' (2010). See www.desmond-project.co.uk.

thinking about it. Be **aware** of what you're eating and when, and always **read the labels**. If a food is high in fat, like a pie, biscuit or pastry, it will contain more calories than eating a piece of fruit instead. When I was a child, my diabetes consultant advised me to eat a tomato when I wanted a packet of crisps. Not much of a swap, I thought. But we do often eat just for the sake of it rather than because we're hungry, or when we need to eat because BG is low.

Smoking

Smoking is addictive so, although you know that it isn't good for your health, it is often a difficult habit to give up. By smoking when you have diabetes, you are increasing your risk of having a heart attack and/or stroke and problems with a reduced blood supply to the legs, increasing your amputation risk. This is because blood vessels become narrowed and furred up so there is less room for blood to reach your brain, heart and legs.

The NHS has said that if you give up smoking, your body will feel the benefit after only 20 minutes, and the longer you don't have a cigarette or tobacco, the better.

Case study: Jim

Jim Jenkins was 50 with Type 2 diabetes. He smoked twenty cigarettes a day for thirty years and was always short of breath. One day he developed chest pains and he went to see his GP. Jim was told that the best thing he could do for his health was to stop smoking and his GP prescribed nicotine replacement patches. Quitting wasn't easy, but Jim has now been a non-smoker for two years. He admits that he still thinks about having a cigarette, but his lowered risk of having a heart attack stops him.

FACT: Smoking and diabetes are a deadly combination. People with diabetes who smoke have an increased risk of premature death and an increased risk of heart disease.

Time period[16]	Benefit to your body when you stop smoking
20 minutes	Your blood pressure and pulse return to normal.
8 hours	Your chances of having a heart attack start to drop.
24 hours	Your lungs start to clear of mucus and waste products.
48 hours	Nicotine is no longer found in the body and your ability to taste and smell improve.
72 hours	Your breathing is easier and your energy levels increase.
2–12 weeks	Blood circulation increases throughout your whole body.
3–9 months	Breathing problems improve as lung function increases by 5–10 per cent.
5 years	Your risk of heart attack is now half that of a smoker.
10 years	Lung cancer risk is half that of a smoker; heart attack risk is similar to a non-smoker.

WORK AND SLEEP

The type of work you do can actually increase your chances of developing Type 2 diabetes as well as playing a role in raising BG levels. Your metabolism – the way your body uses energy – is disrupted by a lack of sleep, so if you are getting less than seven hours per night or your sleep is often disrupted, the insulin your own body produces (if you do not have diabetes or you have Type 2) works less well to reduce BG because of a hormonal imbalance.

16 What happens when you quit? (2018). See www.nhs.uk/smokefree/why-quit/what-happens-when-you-quit.

The continual release of the hormones *epinephrine* and *cortisol* when you can't sleep stresses the body and this prevents the immune system working efficiently.[17] Epinephrine and cortisol stop other hormones, such as insulin and *serotonin* – the hormone that makes us feel happy – from working properly and, over time, this can lead to illnesses like depression, heart disease, hardening of the arteries, Type 2 diabetes and certain cancers.

FACT: Insulin is 25 per cent less effective at lowering BG levels in people without diabetes who have had disrupted sleep over three nights. If you have Type 1 or Type 2 diabetes and sleep problems, this could be a reason you have poor BG control and a high HbA1c.

Overwhelming evidence has shown a link between a lack of sleep and the development of Type 2 diabetes.[18] During a normal period of seven to eight hours' undisrupted sleep, the body is not expecting food. If sleep is disrupted or sleeping patterns change entirely – such as during shift work – there's an increase in *insulin insensitivity*, where insulin doesn't work as well and more and more is produced to reduce BG. Insulin insensitivity starts before the development of Type 2 diabetes. People who sleep during the day and work at night are often found to have insulin insensitivity because shift work causes another hormone, *melatonin*, to be released at the wrong times. Melatonin stops insulin working properly, causing higher BG levels when a person doing shift work eats something. This is not the same as Type 2 diabetes – it's the way the body reacts to sleep deprivation or shift work *before* Type 2 develops.

17 Wax, R. (2013), *Sane New World: Taming the Mind* (Croydon: Hodder & Stoughton).
18 Francesco, P. et al. (2010), 'Quantity and quality of sleep and incidence of Type 2 diabetes', *Diabetes Care* 33(2), pp.414–20.

SEX

Unfortunately, having diabetes can have a big impact on your sex life if your BG control is not good.

There is very little information available about reduced sex drive in women with diabetes (most research has focused on *erectile dysfunction*). High glucose levels cause dryness of the mouth and vagina, thrush infections, and can be the cause of an irregular menstrual cycle. A low or non-existent sex drive may be owing to psychological issues like poor self-esteem. If you have any problems with this area of your life, it is important to speak to your doctor or diabetes specialist who can refer you to a counsellor or psychologist specially trained in diabetes-related issues.

ISSUES FOR WOMEN

In terms of fertility, women can find it difficult to become pregnant if their HbA1c and general diabetes control is poor. If you are planning to become pregnant you should consult your GP and/or your diabetes care team – they can help you to achieve the best possible BG control to enable a healthy conception and pregnancy. Pregnancy for diabetic mothers is definitely more complicated than for mothers without the condition. Your GP, midwife and diabetes care team will be aware of this and may suggest you have your baby in one of the specialised birthing centres around the country that can provide up-to-date technology and expertise.

FACT: If the mother already has diabetes, the child is six times more likely to develop it.

> **FACT:** If you have Type 1 diabetes and become pregnant, your insulin needs will change. If you have Type 2 diabetes, you will be advised to stop taking glucose-reducing tablets and change to insulin injections while pregnant. You should be able to return to tablets after the birth. If gestational diabetes develops while you're pregnant, you will be advised to reduce your carbohydrate intake and you may need to take insulin until you have the baby.

Pregnancy and Type 1 diabetes

If you have Type 1 diabetes and become pregnant your insulin needs will double or even treble. This need usually begins to fall several weeks before the birth. Then, in the last week or fortnight, you will actually become hypo more often. When your baby is born, your insulin requirements will fall dramatically as your BG eventually returns to pre-pregnancy levels. You will be advised to eat less carbohydrate after the birth and to regularly monitor your BG levels, so insulin needs will be reduced.

If you already suffer from diabetic eye disease – retinopathy – and the condition is severe, this may get worse while you are pregnant. This is also a possibility if you make drastic improvements to your BG control because you are pregnant. This worsening of diabetic retinopathy is ironically due to improved BG levels in blood reaching the tiny blood capillaries in the eyes. This situation reverses when your baby is born and your eyesight becomes the same as it was before your pregnancy. Diabetic kidney damage – nephropathy – may also become worse during pregnancy, but this situation usually reverses after the birth.[19]

19 Jarvis, S. & Rubin, A. (2003), *Diabetes for Dummies* (Chichester: John Wiley & Sons, Ltd.), pp.96–7.

FACT: If the mother had high BG levels and ketones during pregnancy the baby may have impaired intelligence as it becomes older.

Pregnancy and Type 2 Diabetes

Women with Type 2 diabetes are more likely to develop high blood pressure when they become pregnant.[20] You will be advised to monitor your BG more frequently during your pregnancy. Most women with Type 2 will be able to go the full term of thirty-nine weeks but if you do have high blood pressure, or you had a previous difficult delivery, you may be advised not to go to full term.

Case study: Gloria

Gloria Sanchez was 35 with Type 2 diabetes for three years before she became pregnant with her fourth child. Gloria was advised by her diabetes team to stop her glucose-reducing medication as it was not good for the baby, and her consultant started Gloria on insulin. She soon got used to testing her BG before and after meals and adjusting her insulin accordingly. Gloria was also given nutrition education by the hospital dietician, who advised her to reduce her daily calories, and to eat smaller meals to even out her BG levels. Just one week later, Gloria's BG tests were within normal range most of the time and she went on to have a healthy, normal-weight baby boy.

20 Jarvis, S. & Rubin, A. (2003), *Diabetes for Dummies* (Chichester: John Wiley & Sons Ltd.), p.97.

Pregnancy and gestational diabetes

Varying BG levels during pregnancy mean that tests to determine gestational diabetes in the mother are often inaccurate; the condition is hard to diagnose and there is no definition of BG level to confirm that someone definitely has gestational diabetes. In a glucose tolerance test where 75g of glucose is given by mouth, a result after two hours that is above 7.8 mmol/L (140.4 mg/dl American measurement) but below 11.1 mmol/L (199.8 mg/dl) is generally accepted as *impaired glucose tolerance.*[21]

A result above 11.1 mmol/L after two hours is diagnosed as *gestational diabetes.* Although BG levels are higher, gestational diabetes develops from the twentieth week of pregnancy. There is less chance of birth defects from hyperglycaemia because the baby's development is more advanced than if the mother has high BG levels from conception.

FACT: 18 per cent of pregnant mothers develop gestational diabetes in their twentieth week.

Issues in early pregnancy

The most important factor when you have diabetes and become pregnant is to have the best possible BG levels. Poor diabetes control at conception and during the first five to nine weeks of the baby's development (often at a time before the woman knows she's pregnant) can cause miscarriages and birth defects. The downside of trying to tighten your BG control is that you may have more hypos because there is less glucose available if you are doing the same activities every day. This is more likely during early pregnancy, but your mild hypos won't harm the baby. **Test your blood glucose levels** throughout the day and also occasionally during the night.

21 Jarvis, S. & Rubin, A. (2003), *Diabetes for Dummies* (Chichester: John Wiley & Sons Ltd.), p.97.

> FACT: Taking 400mcg of folic acid daily from a month before you conceive to twelve weeks into your pregnancy helps your baby's spinal cord to develop normally.

Late pregnancy

During the later stages of pregnancy, larger babies are the main problem for mothers with diabetes. Large is defined as 4.5kg or above at birth. When a non-diabetic mother has a large baby, its development is in line with its size but, as we've seen, large babies born to diabetic mothers are not fully matured. If diabetes is undiagnosed and BG levels are not reduced, the risk of birth defects is high as excess glucose causes areas of the baby where fat is stored to become enlarged. The baby will generally lose this excess weight during the first year but there is an increased risk of becoming obese from age six to eight years.[22]

> FACT: Having poor BG control during pregnancy can mean the baby becomes abnormally large because its pancreas is producing insulin to reduce BG – this causes a high amount of fat to be stored in its shoulders, chest, abdomen, arms and legs. Large babies are delivered early, although they're not full term. Controlling your BG can prevent your child becoming obese or even developing diabetes themselves.

22 Jarvis, S. & Rubin, A. (2003), *Diabetes for Dummies* (Chichester: John Wiley & Sons Ltd.), pp.101–104.

ISSUES FOR MEN

Erectile dysfunction

Men with diabetes may have problems because of erectile dysfunction. Although this is something that you may not want to talk about, more than half of men with diabetes say they have problems with sexual function and for those over the age of 70, this increases to more than three-quarters of older men with the condition. This is not just a problem seen in men with diabetes – one in ten men *without* diabetes also suffer in this way. Your diabetes may not be to blame though as there are several reasons why a man cannot get and sustain an erection[23]:

- If you smoke, drink alcohol, and/or take illegal drugs such as cannabis.
- If you suffer an accident that affects your penis (you have scar tissue).
- If you have hormonal problems such as too little *testosterone* or too much *prolactin*.
- You have nerve damage due to surgery to your prostate gland, bowels or bladder.
- You have poor blood supply to the penis due to *peripheral vascular disease*.
- You have psychological problems such as anxiety, depression or stress.
- You have suffered spinal cord damage.

Poor BG control over many years can lead to nerve damage so a man cannot have or sustain an erection. Nerve damage happens for the following reasons:

- BG control that is not within normal limits – ideally between 5.0 and 7.0 mmol/L. The worse your BG control, the greater the risk of nerve damage.

23 Jarvis, S. & Rubin, A. (2003), *Diabetes for Dummies* (Chichester: John Wiley & Sons Ltd.), p.104.

- The length of time you've had diabetes has an impact – the longer you've had it, the more likely it is that you will have erectile problems.

Treatments

Luckily for men with diabetes, treatments are available for erectile dysfunction. Both *Viagra* and *Levitra* have been designed specifically to improve blood flow to the penis. These drugs have a 70-per-cent success rate, but they do have some side effects[24], such as headaches, flushing of the face and indigestion. Other effects are having a hint of colour in your vision, blurring of eyesight, and increased sensitivity to light. These problems tend to get better the longer the drugs are used. A third drug, *Uprima* – prescribed for angina, low blood pressure and heart failure – can be dissolved under the tongue and is effective after twenty minutes. Side effects of Uprima are nausea, headaches, dizziness, yawning, not being able to sleep, sweating, flushing of the skin and an altered taste sensation.

> **FACT:** Viagra, Levitra or Uptima should not be taken with nitrate drugs prescribed for chest pain as this may cause a sudden and potentially fatal drop in blood pressure.

- It is also possible for a man to inject his penis to relax the blood vessels and allow more blood to enter. This can only be done two to three times a week.
- A small pill called *Alprostadil* can be inserted via a tube into the opening of the penis after which the tube is removed. This can be used twice in twenty-four hours.

24 www.healthline.com/health/erectile-dysfunction-medications-common-side-effects

- Devices that fit over the penis to create pressure allow blood to enter the tissues. A rubber band is then placed around the base of the penis to retain the blood and this can be kept in place for thirty minutes. Some pain and numbness may occur.
- Penis implants can be used if none of the above alternatives appeal. However, as the result is a permanent erection, a man can have an inflatable device containing fluid implanted into the scrotum so that he can inflate his penis when desired.

FACT: If you have diabetes you will be eligible for any of these remedies for erectile dysfunction on the NHS. If your GP writes 'SLS' on your prescription, the prescription will be issued free of charge.[25]

---

25 Jarvis, S. & Rubin, A. (2003), *Diabetes for Dummies* (Chichester: John Wiley & Sons Ltd.), p.108.

Chapter 7

GETTING BACK CONTROL – MANAGING DIABETES AND SELF-MEDICATION

'I used to be on tablets, but I now take insulin and I feel great!'

You will already have gathered from the case studies in other chapters that there are several treatment options available depending on the type of diabetes you have. Type 1 diabetes is treated with insulin, which can be introduced into the body by injection, insulin pen or insulin pump. People with Type 2 diabetes may be able to control their condition with diet and exercise; diet alone; exercise and BG-lowering medication; or have to move from tablets to insulin if they become pregnant or if the tablets no longer control BG levels as well as they used to.

INSULIN INJECTIONS AND INSULIN PENS

Insulin is used to control BG levels in Type 1 diabetes where the body no longer produces it, or in Type 2 diabetes where the body no longer properly uses the insulin it makes, and tablets cannot control BG. Insulin works by moving glucose from the blood into the body tissues, so it can be used for energy. Insulin also stops the liver from producing even more unnecessary glucose. Some types of insulin work very quickly and others work over many hours.

RAPID-ACTING INSULIN: Humalog; Novolog; Apidra – taken before meals to cover the associated BG rise. This is used with *long-acting insulin* and it takes 10–30 minutes to reach the bloodstream where it works for three to five hours.

SHORT-ACTING INSULIN: Regular (R) insulin is taken 30 minutes before a meal to cover the associated rise in BG. This is used with long-acting insulin and takes 30 minutes to one hour to reach the bloodstream, where it works for twelve hours.

INTERMEDIATE-ACTING INSULIN (NPH): This covers the BG rise when rapid-acting insulin stops working. It is usually taken twice a day with rapid or short-acting insulin, taking ninety minutes to four hours to reach the bloodstream where it works for up to twenty-four hours.

LONG-ACTING INSULIN: Lantus and Levemir – usually combined with rapid or short-acting insulin. It reaches the bloodstream after forty minutes to four hours where it works for up to twenty-four hours.

FACT: It's easier if you *write down* when you should take your insulin and how much.

Insulin comes in vials – small bottles – for use in syringes and insulin pumps, and pre-filled devices or cartridges to use with insulin pens. It is important to **always check** when you receive your prescription to make sure it is the right type and that you have been given the right things you need to take it (syringes or needles). I never used to do this and trusted the pharmacist to get it right until one day I found that a receptionist at my GP surgery had ordered me insulin pen cartridges instead of vials of insulin. Luckily, I had enough insulin to cover me until I picked up the right prescription.

You will be taught how to draw up and inject insulin or how to use an insulin pen when you are first diagnosed with Type 1, or when your consultant decides you need insulin if you have Type 2 diabetes.

FACT: You should never re-use or share needles or syringes. Put used 'sharps' in a puncture-proof container and ask your GP or pharmacist how you can dispose of this.

Case study: Rajesh

Rajesh Karamel had Type 2 diabetes and his consultant told him he needed to take insulin because his tablets weren't bringing his BG down as well as they used to. He needed both short- and long-acting insulin and had to learn how to mix the two in one syringe for injection. He was advised to always draw up the cloudy, long-acting insulin into the syringe first before the clear, short-acting insulin. After Rajesh had done this a few times it became second nature to take his insulin instead of a tablet.

THE DOS AND DON'TS OF INSULIN[1]

- DO store insulin in the fridge – it is a protein, like cheese.
- DO always check your insulin before you inject it. Regular insulin, such as Humalin R or Novoin R, should be clear and colourless like water.
- DO warm the insulin to room temperature between your hands before injecting it.
- DO shake or rotate insulin to mix it before drawing it up if you are told to do so.
- DON'T use Regular insulin if it looks cloudy, thick or coloured, or if there are bits floating in it. N.B.: NPH insulin – such as Humalin N; Novolin N; or pre-mixed insulin containing NPH such as Humalin

1 www.healthline.com/health/type2diabetes/insulin-dos-and-donts

70/30 or Novolin 70/30 – **should** look cloudy or milky after they are mixed.

- DON'T use any kind of NPH insulin if there are bits floating in the mixture or solid white particles stuck to the bottom or sides of the bottle.
- DON'T use insulin that is past the expiry date printed on the outer packaging.
- DON'T ever mix fast- and slow-acting insulin in a syringe unless you are told to by your diabetes consultant or nurse.

Injection sites

> **FACT:** Insulin injected into muscle works more quickly than injecting into fat.

Insulin can be injected beneath the skin into the backs of your upper arms, thighs, abdomen or buttocks (it's not so easy to inject yourself here, though, as you can't see what you're doing). Take care not to inject your insulin in the same place every time because it doesn't work as well and the area may become a fatty lump. For example, use your upper arm in the morning and thigh in the evening. If you do inject in the same area, do it at least 1cm from your previous injection site. **Never** inject insulin into skin where there is a scar or a mole.

> **FACT:** You cannot take insulin by mouth because, as a protein, insulin is broken down by digestion.

Case study: Sharon

Sharon Benson had been injecting insulin for her Type 1 diabetes for five years, although she had a severe needle phobia. Her GP suggested that she try an insulin inhaler to deliver insulin directly to her lungs so it could enter her bloodstream. This treatment wasn't widely available on the NHS, but Sharon's doctor agreed this was a special case. Sharon was excited to try this new way of taking insulin and, because she had never smoked and did not have asthma, she was told it would make a real improvement to her diabetes control. When Sharon tried the insulin inhaler there were a few problems, like a sore throat, cough and some hypos, but she preferred it to taking injections and has now been giving herself insulin this way for six months. She says that it makes her feel liberated and free.

INSULIN PUMPS

Insulin pump therapy has been around since the 1970s and is a different way of getting insulin under the skin. This happens through a small tube – *cannula* – inserted inside a needle. The tube is connected to a reservoir – syringe – of insulin that fits inside the pump. This is renewed and refilled every couple of days, or when BG levels start to rise because the fat under the skin around the insulin infusion site – where the insulin goes in – becomes over-absorbed with insulin so it can't work properly. The pump delivers a continuous background rate – the *basal rate* – of fast-acting insulin and can be programmed to give a larger dose – *bolus* – of insulin to cover the rise in BG when you eat. For some people, an insulin pump helps achieve much better control of BG levels than with injected insulin because the dosages delivered are set according to need during the day and night.

> **FACT:** Insulin pump therapy is also known as CSII – Continuous Subcutaneous Insulin Infusion; IPT; pump therapy; insulin infusion therapy; and intensive insulin treatment.

An insulin pump is battery-driven and is about the size of a pager – 9cm by 5cm – with an area for the reservoir – syringe – of insulin to be inserted when connected to a thin plastic tube. This *infusion set* is inserted into the fat under the skin by the pump user – this doesn't hurt. The pump can also be connected to a continuous glucose sensor, which measures the glucose level in the liquid part of the blood – plasma – every ten minutes. This is especially useful for managing frequent and unexplained hypos – meaning that there's no reason why they happen – and for people with absent or very reduced hypo symptoms.

The pump comes in a range of colours and styles and is made by several different medical companies so there is plenty of choice, although they all do the same job. Pump therapy is sometimes started as soon as a person is diagnosed with Type 1 diabetes in the UK as erratic swings in BG level can be managed much more easily this way than with multiple daily injections – MDI – of insulin. Pump therapy is especially useful for controlling BG levels:

- When there is hypoglycaemia unawareness.
- In children.
- In women who want to conceive or who are pregnant.
- In people with brittle – difficult-to-manage – Type 1 diabetes.

Not surprisingly, an insulin pump is expensive if you want to buy one yourself, costing around £2,500, plus £800 a year for the tubing (insulin infusion sets), plus the syringes and batteries that go with it. For people with Type 1 diabetes that's difficult to control and for some people with Type 2 who are taking insulin, the Department of Health will fund this treatment. If it's felt that you have a **clinical need** for pump therapy because you are unable to manage your diabetes well with multiple daily insulin injections, and/or you have developed some chronic complications because of this, your diabetes consultant will write a letter to your local medical funding committee: the CCG (County Commissioning Group). This will put the case to show you have a clinical need for the treatment because your diabetes cannot be managed effectively any other way.

The real benefit of using a pump is that good control of BG levels can be achieved to prevent or manage any complications that develop through long-term high or poor BG levels. In some countries in Europe, pump therapy is automatically started as soon as a person is diagnosed with Type 1 because the cost of treating chronic diabetic complications – *cataract* surgery and/or kidney dialysis, for example – costs far more than funding pump treatment.

FACT: A pump cannot just be 'plugged in' and forgotten about – the user receives intensive training about how to use this technology properly and effectively.

The user has to know exactly how to get the best out of pump therapy and must be prepared to 'intensively self-manage' their diabetes with frequent BG tests to give the right amount of insulin at the right times. Additionally, a Continuous Glucose Monitoring sensor may also be inserted under the skin and is then attached to a small transmitter that sends glucose results every ten minutes to the pump so the user is warned if BG is going too high or too low. This is very useful if you no longer have warning signs of hypos, especially during the night.

FACT: There are several different makes of insulin pump on the market that all work in the same way. They are all equally good!

Case study: Daniel

Daniel Morgan was 8 years old when his mum, Kelly, first told his diabetes consultant about the difficulties she was having controlling Daniel's BG levels during the night. The consultant felt that an insulin pump would be the answer – providing measured doses of insulin throughout the night, rather than one injected dose working all at once to cause Daniel's night-time hypos and early morning high BGs. Kelly worried that Daniel would not adapt to using the pump – that it might be damaged or become disconnected when he ran around in the playground with his friends at school. The consultant assured Kelly that pumps are made from the same material as crash helmets and that the insulin infusion set is taped on to the skin of the abdomen, so was unlikely to pull out. A fortnight later, Kelly and Daniel were shown how to use the pump by the diabetes nurse. Daniel's now been successfully using his 'insulin box' for six months – he no longer has low and high BG swings during the night.

Case study: Anna

Anna Chatterjee was 24 with poor BG control when she decided to try for a baby. Her consultant advised that her Type 1 diabetes would be much better managed if she used an insulin pump because her dosages could be tailored to her needs if she was prepared to do regular BG tests. Anna wanted her baby to be as healthy as possible and began using a pump to deliver her insulin three months before she conceived. Her HbA1c tests remained constantly within normal range throughout Anna's pregnancy and she had a 2.5kg baby girl without any problems. Because she had been able to improve her BG control so much by using an insulin pump, Anna's consultant agreed she should continue to use it to manage her diabetes effectively.

Advantages of insulin pump therapy over insulin injections or pens:

- An insulin dosage – bolus – can be taken just before a meal or over several hours following a meal if there is slow stomach emptying – determined by medical tests.
- Dosage adjustments of background – basal – insulin help avoid BG swings.
- A bolus of insulin can be given for an unplanned meal or snacks, and meals don't have to be eaten at certain times.
- The pump can be easily disconnected to take a shower or bath.
- There's a safety feature where a maximum dose can be set to prevent insulin overdose.

Disadvantages of pump use:

- A pump is worn on the outside of the body and this shows other people you have diabetes, although it's the size of a pager.
- Pumps are not waterproof so have to be removed when bathing or swimming.
- The insulin in the reservoir can warm up so it doesn't lower BG as well in very hot weather.

FACT: Using insulin pump therapy is an intensive insulin treatment. This means that you have to be prepared to test your BG numerous times a day, be willing to act on the results and use technology to fine-tune your diabetes self-management to be as good as it can be.

GLUCOSE-LOWERING TABLETS

There are many glucose-lowering medications available to treat and manage Type 2 diabetes[2]:

Medication name	When to take it	Effects
BIGUANIDES Metformin – Glucophage. Metformin liquid – Riomet. Metformin extended release – Glucophage XR; Foramet; Glumetza.	Taken twice a day with breakfast and evening meal. Usually taken once a day in the morning.	Bloating, wind, diarrhoea, upset stomach, loss of appetite in first few weeks of taking. Take with food to reduce these effects. Unlikely to cause low BG. There may be lactic acid acidosis in people with reduced kidney and liver function.
SULPHONYLUREAS Glimepiride – Amaryl. Glyburide – Diabeta Micronase. Glipizide – Glucotrol Glucotrol XL. Micronized Glyburide – Glynase.	Taken twice a day with meals.	These stimulate insulin production and can cause low BG, so carry glucose tablets with you. Follow your meal and exercise plan and tell your GP if you have consistently low BG. If your activity increases or your weight decreases, your dose may need to be lowered.
MEGLITINIDES Repagunide – Prandin; D-Phenylalanine derivatives. Nanteglinide – Starlix.	Taken once a day at same time each day.	Works quickly and stops working quickly. May cause low BG but less likely to do so than sulphonylureas.
THIAZOLIDINES Pioglitazone – TZD. Pioglitazone – Actos.	Taken once a day at same time each day.	Swelling/fluid retention. These tablets increase the amount of glucose taken up by muscles, and stop glucose overproduction by the liver, but don't cause low BG. May improve blood fat levels. Increases risk of congestive heart failure in people at risk.

2   Chadhury, A., et al. (2017), 'Clinical review of antidiabetic drugs: implications for Type 2 diabetes mellitus management', *Frontiers of Endocrinology* 8(6). Doi: 10.3389/fendo.2017.00006

DPP-4 INHIBITORS Sitagliptin – Januvia. Saxagliptin – Oxglyza. Linaglyptin – Tradienta.	Take one a day at the same time each day.	Stomach discomfort, diarrhoea, stuffy nose, sore throat, upper respiratory infection. Does not cause low BG and can be taken with Metformin, a sulphony-lurea or Actos.
ALPHA-GLUCOSIDASE INHIBITORS Acarbose – Precose. Miglitol – Glyset.	Take with first bite of your meal; if not eating, don't take.	Slows absorption of carbs into the bloodstream. Can initially cause wind, diarrhoea, abdominal pain. Take with meals to limit a rise in BG after meals. These do not cause low BG.
BILE ACID SEQUESTRANTS Colesevelam – Welchol.	Take once or twice a day with meals. Works with diabetes medication to lower BG. May interact with contraceptives, glyburide, levothyroxine – take thyroid medication and glyburide 4 hours before Welchol.	Constipation, headache, wind, diarrhoea, nausea, heartburn. Used to lower cholesterol. Tell your GP if you have high blood fats or stomach problems, or if you have effects from these tablets that don't go away.
COMBINATION PILLS Pioglitazone & Metformin. Actoplus Met. Glyburide & Metformin – Glucovance. Glipizide & Metformin – Metaglip. Sitagliptin & Metformin – Janumet. Saxagliptin & Metformin – Kombiglyze. Repaglinide & Metformin – Prandimet. Pioglitazone & Glimerpiride – Duetact.	Usually taken once a day; combines the action of each tablet.	Side effects are same as each pill and combin-ation may cause low BG. Combination may reduce number of pills you take.

OTHER INFORMATION YOU SHOULD KNOW

BG-lowering tablets do this in different ways and some of these medications can have side effects. One of the first diabetes medications you may be given for Type 2 are any of the *sulphonylureas* listed. These may cause rashes and weight gain and you may also reach a point where they fail to reduce your BG[3], even if you increase the dose. If this happens, your consultant will reduce your dose back to the level where it was working well.

Metformin can cause an upset stomach, although this improves if the tablets are taken with food. Other possible effects are weight loss and while you might be happy about this, it is owing to nausea and diarrhoea, often accompanied by a poor appetite for food. Intestinal disturbances may also lead to poor absorption of vitamin B12[4], which helps keep your blood and nervous system healthy. You may be advised not to take Metformin if you have poor kidney or liver function, or if you are pregnant/nursing; you will be put onto insulin. Taking Metformin with the indigestion medication *Cimetidine* can increase the amount of Metformin working in the body.[5] You will be advised to stop taking Metformin for a couple of days if you are having surgery or an X-ray involving the injection of dye.

Acarbose should not be taken during pregnancy (insulin will be prescribed to you instead); if you suffer from inflammatory bowel disease, such as Crohn's disease or ulcerative colitis, or if you have reduced liver or kidney function, a hernia or if you have previously had abdominal surgery.

Glitazones work best on BG after eating because they are quickly absorbed; improve insulin resistance, and reduce the amount of insulin the body has to produce to reduce BG. These tablets take two to three months before they start working to full effect, so they are usually taken with another medication such as Metformin to reduce BG. This can lead to a weight gain of 1–4kg over the first six months of taking them. They can also cause fluid retention in the lower legs (*oedema*) and iron deficiency (anaemia). Cases of improved fertility and unexpected pregnancy have been reported! These tablets should

3   Jarvis, S. & Rubin, A. (2003), *Diabetes For Dummies* (Chichester: John Wiley & Sons Ltd.), p.177.

4   Ibid., p.180.

5   Maideen, N. M. P. (2017), 'Drug interactions of Metformin involving drug transporter proteins', *Advanced Pharmacology Bulletin* 7(4), pp. 501–505.

NOT be taken by people with poor liver or kidney function, or by pregnant or breastfeeding mothers.[6]

Meglitinides are broken down by the liver so if you have poor liver function, the dose of these tablets will be reduced. If liver disease is advanced, you will be advised **not** to take Meglitinides. If you have kidney impairment, your GP and diabetes consultant should carefully monitor any increase in the dose. These tablets sometimes cause a rash to develop, and/or a stomach upset and vomiting in the case of allergy to this medication. Pregnant and breastfeeding women, people under 18 or over 75 and people with severe liver disease should **not** take Meglitinides.

6   Jarvis, S. & Rubin, A. (2003), *Diabetes for Dummies* (Chichester: John Wiley & Sons Ltd.), pp.184–5.

Chapter 8

Know Your Enemy! – Understanding Diabetic Complications

'Keeping complications at bay is my biggest motivation.'

The reason for trying to get the best possible BG control is to avoid or delay the development of long-term complications. You may have heard the word 'complications' a few times in connection with diabetes, especially if you have had no symptoms of Type 2 diabetes and have been living with high BG levels for a few years. Unfortunately, serious medical problems can happen whatever type of diabetes you have, and these may take up to ten years to appear after a period of poor BG control.

> **FACT: You can do a lot to reduce your risk of developing the complications of diabetes.**

How do complications start?

When BG levels are high, your blood becomes thick like syrup so your heart has to work much harder to pump blood around the body. The glucose in your blood sticks to the sides of blood vessels, narrowing the amount of space available for your blood to flow through. The amount of glucose that attaches to your red blood cells over three months – the life span of these cells – is measured in an HbA1c test. Glucose can also attach itself to white blood cells and other substances in the blood, so glucose levels higher than anything up to the normal 6.0 per cent – 42 mmol/L – can change the function of cells. Red blood cells are unable to hold as much oxygen; white blood cells are not as able to fight infection.

These changes in cell function start the development of complications. Another abnormal process in the body occurs when it's trying to use glucose as fuel, but there is too much, so the excess glucose instead breaks down into harmful toxins. Body cells also shrivel up because the water balance inside and outside the cell is affected. Genetic factors may also cause complications.

FACT: One in six NHS beds is currently taken up by a person with Type 1 or Type 2 diabetes and complications.

What kinds of complications are there?

The first complications of poor BG control you may see are eye, nerve and/or kidney problems. Smaller blood vessels, such as those at the back of the eyes, become weaker and may leak or burst. Larger blood vessels that supply your heart, brain and legs are also more likely to become blocked.

High amounts of glucose do not just cause problems with blood vessels – they also affect your nerves, particularly the ones in your feet. But the good news is… diabetic complications are **not** inevitable.

Kidneys

Elevated amounts of glucose in your blood and urine can damage your kidneys as they try to filter out the excess. Glucose molecules are large, disrupting the structures that cleanse the blood as they pass through urine filtration membranes within the kidneys. These thicken and expand into the space occupied by the small blood vessels. Because diabetic kidney disease – *nephropathy* – is not painful, damage can go undetected for many years. After fifteen years, the problem may become severe. Blood tests can show major kidney malfunction after twenty years and the kidneys may fail entirely[1]. But don't panic!

First, glucose is present in the urine only when your BG reaches 10 mmol/L or above.

Second, your GP and/or diabetes consultant will ask you to provide a urine sample at least every year. This is tested for the presence of small amounts of protein – the first stage of kidney disease. If this is found you will be prescribed medication to slow the progression of the disease.

Third, tightening BG control is the best way to tackle or prevent the first stage of diabetic kidney disease.

Other factors that are known to contribute to kidney damage are high blood pressure; high blood fats such as cholesterol; genetic factors such as ethnicity; and smoking.

Eyes

Having diabetes can affect your eyes in several ways[2], again because of higher-than-normal BG levels.

CATARACTS happen when the lens of the eyes develop opaque areas that can block vision. These develop far more often in people with diabetes of all ages than in the non-diabetic population. When a cataract is mature it is surgically removed; a plastic lens is implanted to replace your own and your sight can be as good as it always was.

1   MacIsaac, R. J. & Watts, G. F. (2005), 'Diabetes and the Kidney'. In K. M. Shaw & M. H. Cummings (eds.), *Diabetes: Chronic Complications*, Second Edition, Chapter 2 (Chichester: John Wiley & Sons Ltd.), pp. 23–6.
2   Shotliff, K. & Duncan, G. (2005), 'Diabetes and the Eye'. In K. M. Shaw & M. H. Cummings (eds.), *Diabetes: Chronic Complications*, Second Edition, Chapter 1 (Chichester: John Wiley & Sons Ltd.), pp.1–19.

GLAUCOMA is a disease where there is increased pressure within the eyes that may damage the optic nerve. It is a common problem in people with diabetes and if it's not checked regularly, it can cause blindness because it destroys the optic nerve. However, eye drops prescribed by your medics can lower this pressure.

RETINOPATHY is the name for diabetic changes to the retina at the back of the eye owing to high BG levels over time. It can cause blindness if left untreated. The first changes are seen after ten years in both Type 1 and Type 2 diabetes. There are different types of retinopathy that are categorised by their potential to cause visual loss[3]:

- Background *retinopathy* – stable but can cause problems.
- Retinal haemorrhages and hard *exudates* – capillary bleeds and leaked yellow fat deposits that cause scarring.
- *Macular oedema* – fluid build-up causing loss of vision.
- Cotton wool spots and soft exudates – decreased blood supply to the nerves and destruction of the nerves of the retina. These changes can go on to become proliferative retinopathy, which, if untreated, causes loss of vision.

You are more likely to develop retinopathy if[4]:

- You are of South Asian origin.
- You have certain genetic factors as well as your diabetes.
- You have high blood pressure.
- You have had diabetes for a long time.
- You smoke or regularly drink alcohol.

3   Shotliff, K. & Duncan, G. (2005), 'Diabetes and the Eye'. In K. M. Shaw & M. H. Cummings (eds.), *Diabetes: Chronic Complications*, Second Edition, Chapter 1 (Chichester: John Wiley & Sons, Ltd.), p.7.
4   Jarvis, S. & Rubin, A. (2003), *Diabetes for Dummies* (Chichester: John Wiley & Sons Ltd.), p.76.

There is no medication you can take for retinopathy, but laser surgery has saved the vision of many people. There are some risks with this procedure though: minor loss of vision owing to burns to the retina, a small reduction in night-time vision and a reduction in the visual field in the treated eye. Eye and kidney disease often go hand in hand.

Case study: Mia

Mia Villano was 34 when she developed proliferative retinopathy and nephropathy within six months of one another. She said her eyesight was like looking through a piece of gauze, although she wasn't aware of her kidney problems because there was no pain or other symptoms. Her consultant told her that eye and kidney problems are also associated with cardiovascular problems. Mia's complications had developed because of repeated bouts of keto-acidosis as a result of very high BG levels as a teenager.

Eye screening

There is a National Screening Programme for Diabetic Retinopathy. If you are over 11 years old with diabetes, you will be offered photographic eye screening every year to check the back of your eyes – the retina. Screening will pick up only diabetic changes in the retina, so it doesn't detect problems like cataracts or glaucoma. In some cases, these problems will be seen during the screening process and you will be referred to the hospital eye clinic directly or to your GP for more checks. It is **very important** to have your eyes screened for diabetic retinopathy because[5]:

- Untreated diabetic retinopathy is one of the major causes of blindness in the working-age population.

5   www.nidirect.gov.uk/articles/diabetic-eye-screening

- If detected early, laser treatment is very effective at reducing sight loss from diabetic retinopathy.
- Diabetic retinopathy does not usually affect your sight until the changes to your retina are fairly advanced. By this stage, laser treatment is less able to reduce sight loss.

Screening your eyes for retinopathy means regular examinations to detect any diabetic changes that could affect your sight. These changes are known as sight-threatening diabetic retinopathy. Screening will decide whether or not you need follow-up treatment from the hospital eye clinic for diabetic retinopathy. If you have no diabetic changes or if your existing retinopathy is stable, you will be asked to come back for screening a year later.

FACT: Everyone over the age of eleven with diabetes needs to have eye screening. This is the case if you take insulin or tablets, or you use diet and exercise to manage your BG levels, and whether you see your GP or a diabetes specialist for your diabetes care.

If you already visit a hospital eye clinic for another eye condition, and then you develop diabetes, the doctor you already see there will take over your eye screening. Make sure this doctor is aware that you have diabetes so they specifically check for diabetic retinopathy each year – hospital clinics tend to have visiting eye specialists with them for a year before they move to another hospital, so you won't get to see the same person each time.

FACT: You will still need to visit your optician up to every two years for sight tests, glasses or contact lenses.

So, what actually happens during retinal screening?

- Your GP, hospital, local retinal screening programme or mobile unit in your area will have your details and are bound by a duty of care and confidentiality.
- You will be sent a letter inviting you to attend a screening appointment. The screening may be at your GP's surgery, your opticians, at the local hospital, or another convenient venue local to you if it's a mobile screening unit.
- The procedure will be explained when you arrive and you can ask any questions you have about the screening.
- They will take a record of your details and your level of sight.
- You will be given eye drops – these sting for a few seconds – which make the pupils of your eyes bigger to allow the retina at the back of the eye to be photographed. After fifteen minutes, your vision will become blurred and it will be difficult to focus on objects near you. This is normal, so don't worry. Your vision will go back to normal again – effects last between two and six hours, depending on which drops you're given. You won't be able to drive yourself home afterwards.
- You will be seated in front of a machine that takes a photograph of the retina of each eye. The camera does not touch your eyes. You will see a flash of light for each photograph taken. The light is bright but this is a painless procedure and you shouldn't feel uncomfortable.

You should take your glasses with you and a pair of sunglasses for afterwards as you will find your eyes are sensitive to light because your pupils have been enlarged. If you wear contact lenses, you will need to remove them so the camera can photograph your retinas – so take your lens container with you. You can put your lenses back in afterwards, but you may want to give your eyes a rest and wear glasses instead, if you have them.

> **FACT:** You should not drive yourself to and from your eye screening appointment.

Very rarely, the eye drops can cause a rapid increase in pressure in the eyes. This only happens in people who are already at risk of developing this problem. If this happens it will be treated quickly in the eye unit. The symptoms of high pressure in the eyes are:

- Pain or severe discomfort in your eyes.
- Redness of the white of your eyes.
- Blurred vision, sometimes with rainbow halos around lights.

> **FACT:** If you experience any of these symptoms after screening you should return to the eye unit or go to the hospital Accident and Emergency department.

After your eye screening your retinal photographs may have to be seen by an eye specialist or more than one health professional, so you won't get the results straightaway. You will be told how long it will be before you get your written results – if you aren't told, be sure to ask. The results will also be sent to your GP and to the National Screening Programme. No one else will see your results unless you give them permission. You may want to take a copy of your screening results to give to your diabetes team. You may be called back to the screening centre if:

- They find sight-threatening retinopathy needing follow-up treatment from the hospital eye clinic.
- The photographs are unclear and don't give an accurate result.
- The level of retinopathy you have needs to be monitored more often than once a year.

- Other eye conditions are found during the screening process that need more investigation.

If you are worried about or have problems with your eyes in between eye screening appointments, don't wait for your next screening appointment – seek professional advice.

The screening unit will keep your photographs for at least eight years so they can compare future ones and detect changes over time. A small number of retinal photographs undergo quality control tests to make sure they have been properly assessed. You can reduce your risk of developing sight-threatening eye changes by:

- Keeping your BG levels within normal range – aim for between 5.0 and 7.0 mmol/L.
- Making sure your blood pressure is monitored regularly.
- Attending regular eye screening appointments.
- Attending regular diabetes checks.
- Having your blood fats – lipids and cholesterol – checked regularly.
- Quitting smoking.

Nerve disease

High BG levels often take their toll on the nervous system in the form of neuropathy – nerve damage – and 60 per cent of people diagnosed with diabetes will experience this. This complication is usually seen in people who have had diabetes for many years, those over forty, and in people who smoke. There are two kinds:

PERIPHERAL NEUROPATHY – affecting the feet and hands.

AUTONOMIC NEUROPATHY – damage to the nerves that control actions we don't have to think about, like breathing, heartbeat, digestive function and bladder function.

Case study: Christina

Christina Santos had both peripheral and autonomic neuropathies because her Type 2 diabetes had been poorly controlled for over twenty years. She described the problems in her lower legs and feet as flashing pains, heavy legs, numbness, extreme sensitivity to touch, and muscle tenderness. She also had no knee or ankle reflexes. She had developed several foot ulcers over the years and amputation had been suggested because of both her nerve damage and poor blood supply. Christina was told that the damage was irreversible, so she continued to eat whatever she liked and did not take her diabetes medication regularly. She also had problems with autonomic neuropathy because of long-term high BG levels. She developed *gastroparesis* – delayed stomach emptying – meaning her food was digested slowly because her stomach didn't empty at the normal rate. This caused problems with high BG levels because Christina's medication was not working when her meals were digested. Christina also suffered other side effects of gastro-intestinal nerve damage such as abdominal bloating, wind, pain and severe diarrhoea.

FACT: A foot ulcer develops in approximately one in six people with diabetes at some time in their life.

You may have tests when you visit your diabetes clinic to see if there are any signs of nerve damage in your feet. These include tests to see if you can feel vibration or temperature changes and testing to see if you can sense something touching your skin. If your consultant finds that you do not feel certain sensations in response to these tests, a diagnosis of peripheral neuropathy will be made. This may be[6]:

SENSORY nerve damage.

MOTOR nerve damage (damage to the nerves that send impulses to the muscles to make them move).

AUTONOMIC nerve damage.

Some people with autonomic neuropathy may not have all of the usual symptoms, and symptoms such as abdominal bloating and diarrhoea can be mistaken for *irritable bowel syndrome*.

Below you can find a list of disorders associated with neuropathy:

Sensation problems

These are very common in people with diabetes and either affect many nerves in the body or only a few. *Distal polyneuropathy* affects many of the nerves in the feet and hands and is caused by high BG levels over time. The symptoms of polyneuropathy are[7]:

- Reduced ability to feel light touch and a lack of awareness of the position of the foot.
- Reduced pain and temperature sensations.
- Tingling and burning sensations.
- Weakness.
- Sensations like walking on pebbles.

6   Meeking, D., Holland, E. & Land, D. (2005), 'Diabetes and Foot Disease'. In K. M. Shaw & M. H. Cummings (eds.), *Diabetes: Chronic Complications*, Second Edition, Chapter 3 (Chichester: John Wiley & Sons, Ltd.), pp. 61–4.
7   Ibid., p. 61.

- Increased sensitivity to touch.
- Loss of balance and/or co-ordination.

These symptoms are often worse during the night.

FACT: There's a medication designed to help with nerve damage symptoms – *Gabapentin*. This reduces neuropathy pain, allowing better sleep.

Case study: David

David Moore was 49, having had Type 1 diabetes for thirty years. Although he had improved his BG control over the past ten years, earlier nerve damage had led to neuropathy in his legs, feet and hands. These areas of his body were numb and cold, although he had a good blood supply in both feet. David tended to walk around the house barefoot and one day, he trod on one of his son's Lego bricks. He felt some discomfort but thought no more of it. A week later David's wife, Lynn, noticed he was limping slightly. She examined his foot and found that a split in the skin on the sole had become infected. Lynn cleaned and dressed the wound. David went to his GP and, to his surprise, was told he would have to go into hospital. Because people with diabetes have slow wound healing, David remained in hospital for two weeks as the wound was intensively treated with antibiotic powder. David was not allowed to walk on the foot for a month and he was discharged from hospital on crutches. He now always makes sure he wears slippers indoors and checks his feet every day.

FOOT ULCERS are a very serious complication that can happen because of loss of feeling in the feet[8]. Normal areas of pressure on the feet cannot be detected as pain and an area of hard skin develops. Over time, this continued pressure on this hardened skin causes it to break down and soften until it becomes mushy and comes away, leaving a deep hole, or ulcer in the foot that becomes infected. If professional help is not sought for a diabetic foot ulcer, the hole grows larger and the blood supply dies off. At this stage, the only thing that can be done is to amputate – possibly the whole lower leg – to save the person's life.

CHARCOT JOINTS – neuroarthropathy. The small foot bones can be moved out of position so multiple pain-free fractures occur. The foot and ankle swell up and become red and the foot eventually becomes useless.[9]

Case study: Eva

Eva Gomez was 29 with Type 1 diabetes that was very difficult to control from age ten. One morning, Eva woke up and the whole of her left foot was swollen to three times that of her right. The foot didn't hurt, and Eva couldn't afford to miss work, so she put on a pair of roomy boots and hobbled to her job. The next day, Eva's foot was no better. She did not have a good relationship with her diabetes consultant because he would warn her about her poor BG control. Eva continued to walk around and, after eighteen months, her foot finally went back to normal size. She was horrified to find

8   Meeking, D., Holland, E. & Land, D. (2005), 'Diabetes and Foot Disease'. In K. M. Shaw & M. H. Cummings (eds.), *Diabetes: Chronic Complications*, Second Edition, Chapter 3. (Chichester: John Wiley & Sons Ltd.), p.49.
9   Ibid., pp.209–10.

that her left foot was now much wider across the bridge than her right. Her big toe had dislocated downwards and her third and fourth toes were now bent and misshapen. She also had a large area of hard skin on her sole beneath the third and fourth toe. Eva now wishes she had gone to see her doctor when she first found her foot was swollen. As she walks, although there is no pain, her left foot makes a crunching sound as the bones grind and Eva can now only wear flat, orthopaedic shoes.

FACT: Good, regular foot care can reduce amputation rates by 45–85 per cent.

Movement problems

Diabetes also affects the nerves and muscles that allow us to move around easily because of changes to their blood supply. Any of our nerves may be affected and unfortunately, the only way to prevent this complication is with good BG control. For those people who have extreme difficulty in achieving good BG results, the best control possible with insulin pump therapy is sometimes not enough to overcome many years of poor BG control, meaning associated nerve damage is inevitable.

Problems caused by poor BG control over time can show themselves in a number of ways:

THE HEART may not pump more blood to the muscles when it's needed, such as when standing up from a sitting position, causing light headedness. The heart rate may also be very fast and/or the heart rhythm may become disrupted, increasing the chance of sudden death.[10] When there is autonomic nerve damage the resting heart rate is high, blood pressure drops very low when standing, and the general heart rate when breathing in and out is low. The heart may also become larger – *cardiomyopathy* – and is unable to pump enough blood, leading to a faster heart rate and problems if there is already a high blood pressure.

CORONARY HEART DISEASE means the blood supply to the heart becomes gradually less and less[11]. This is owing to narrowing of the coronary arteries supplying the heart and this is something that happens over time in people with Type 1 diabetes. Heart disease occurs much sooner in people with Type 2 diabetes because BG levels can be abnormally high for as long as twelve years before diagnosis[12]. Meanwhile, high BG levels cause the arteries to fur up and become narrow.

Other factors that increase the risk of heart disease in Type 2 diabetes or pre-diabetes – before Type 2 is diagnosed:

- Having high blood pressure.
- High blood fats – such as cholesterol.
- Insulin resistance – also known as pre-diabetes – BG concentrations higher than normal, but lower than established limits for diabetes itself.
- Obesity, especially fat around the waist.
- Smoking.

VASCULAR DISEASE occurs when the blood vessels in the hands and feet

10 Fisher, M. & Shaw, K. (2005), 'Diabetes and the Heart'. In K. M. Shaw & M. H. Cummings (eds.), *Diabetes: Chronic Complications*, Second Edition, Chapter 6. (Chichester: John Wiley & Sons Ltd.), p.122.

11 Ibid., p.122.

12 Diabetes UK (2008), *Early Identification of Type 2 Diabetes and the new Vascular Risk Assessment and Management Programme*. Position Statement Update. (London: Diabetes UK.)

become blocked – this happens at an earlier age in people with diabetes than in the general population who do not have diabetes. Because of vascular disease, after a decade, one-third of people with diabetes will have lost the arterial pulses in their feet[13]. This complication of diabetes affects multiple arteries in the body and this may happen because of things you can't do anything about, such as genetic factors; becoming older; and having diabetes. But there are things you can do to slow down this damage to the main blood vessels:

- Reducing your HbA1c level.
- Stopping smoking.
- Reducing your blood cholesterol level.
- Managing high blood pressure levels.
- Controlling your body weight.

THE BRAIN: If the arteries supplying the brain with oxygen become blocked there are serious consequences. A partial restriction in blood supply – *transient ischaemia* – results in a mini-stroke with slurring of speech, muscle weakness down one side of the body, and numbness[14]. This frightening situation may last for a few minutes, hours or days depending on how much of the artery is blocked. If the artery closes completely owing to the formation of a large blood clot, a full stroke occurs. The good news is, the quicker a stroke sufferer gets professional help, the sooner treatment to dissolve the blood clot can be given. This is the reason that people with diabetes are prescribed a daily 75mg dose of aspirin to thin the blood and prevent clots.

THE LARGE INTESTINE can be affected dramatically by autonomic neuropathy, where there is ongoing and frequent diarrhoea, and loss of bowel

---

13 Meeking, D., Holland, E. & Land, D. (2005), 'Diabetes and Foot Disease'. In K. M. Shaw & M. H. Cummings (eds.), *Diabetes: Chronic Complications*, Second Edition, Chapter 3 (Chichester: John Wiley & Sons Ltd.), p.54.

14 Cranston, I. (2005), 'Diabetes and the Brain'. In K. M. Shaw & M. H. Cummings (eds.), *Diabetes: Chronic Complications*. Second Edition, Chapter 7 (Chichester: John Wiley & Sons Ltd.), p.147.

control[15]. This can be treated with medication to stop the need for such frequent visits to the toilet, but there may also be alternate diarrhoea and constipation. If the stomach nerves are damaged, the time taken to digest food slows down, causing problems with matching BG-lowering dosages with BG working times. Insulin pump therapy helps match rates of digestion to insulin needs in Type 1 diabetes and a medication called *Metoclopramide* helps the stomach to empty more quickly.

THE GALL BLADDER can develop gallstones owing to nerve damage so that it doesn't empty properly after eating, especially if the meal has a high fat content. Bile – produced by the body to break down fat – builds up and hardens in the gall bladder to form gall stones.

BLADDER nerves become damaged, causing loss of awareness of when the bladder is full. This leads to urinary tract infections, urine does not flow normally but dribbles out, and a person with this problem may have to strain to push urine out of the bladder. Medication can increase the force of the bladder muscles when they contract to release urine and attempting to urinate every four hours can help to avoid infections.[16]

SEXUAL FUNCTION problems are experienced by 50 per cent of men with diabetes (erectile dysfunction) and 30 per cent of women (vaginal dryness).[17]

THE PUPILS OF THE EYES contain nerves that may be affected by autonomic neuropathy so they cannot adjust to let in more or less light when needed.

15 Murray, C. & Emmanuel, A. (2005), 'Diabetes and the Gastrointestinal System'. In K. M. Shaw & M. H. Cummings (eds.), *Diabetes: Chronic Complications,* Second Edition, Chapter 8 (Chichester: John Wiley & Sons Ltd.), p.169.
16 Jarvis, S. & Rubin, A. (2003), *Diabetes for Dummies* (Chichester: John Wiley & Sons Ltd.), p.83.
17 Cummings, M. H. (2005), 'Diabetes and Sexual Health'. In K. M. Shaw & M. H. Cummings (eds.), *Diabetes: Chronic Complications,* Second Edition, Chapter 5. (Chichester: John Wiley & Sons Ltd.), pp.95–115.

Case study: Dev

Dev Mobarak was in his mid-40s with Type 2 diabetes when he began experiencing severe shoulder pain, limited movement and stiffness. His GP diagnosed a frozen shoulder and sent Dev for intense physiotherapy to loosen the joint and reduce the pain. Dev found these physio sessions incredibly painful and sought a second opinion with a private doctor specialising in joint conditions. Dev was diagnosed with *shoulder adhesive capsulitis* and he was told this was a complication caused by very high BG levels over time. It limited the movement in his arm because the surface of the shoulder joint had thickened and connective tissue had stuck to the head of the humerus bone. The physiotherapy Dev had been doing during his misdiagnosis had pulled the abnormal connections in his shoulder, causing more pain. Dev improved his BG control and found the pain was reduced, although the adhesions were permanent, so he was left with limited movement.

OTHER CONSEQUENCES OF LIVING WITH DIABETES are joint and muscle pain. This is because diabetes affects all body systems, including muscle and bone. Some joint conditions are similar to problems experienced by the general population, making them difficult to confirm as diabetes-related:

THE HANDS of people with diabetes may become stiff, painful and swollen, reducing movement as the small bones are affected. This is seen in 50 per cent of people with Type 1 or Type 2 diabetes.[18] *Carpal tunnel syndrome* – where the tendons in the hands and wrists shorten so the fingers rest in a claw-like position is very common in association with diabetes, as is *Dupuytren's disease*

---

18 Browne, D. L. & McCrae, F. C. (2005), 'Diabetes and Musculoskeletal Disease'. In K. M. Shaw & M. H. Cummings (eds.), *Diabetes: Chronic Complications*, Second Edition, Chapter 9 (Chichester: John Wiley & Sons Ltd.), p.206.

– where the tendons of the wrist shorten and the palms become thickened so they cannot be placed together in a prayer-like position.

THE VERTEBRA – spinal joints – may join together in a condition known as *hyperostosis*, limiting movement in obese people with Type 2 diabetes. Gout and *osteoarthritis* are common in the bones of the feet, especially in association with obesity where the feet have to support a greater weight. A condition where there's lack of bone mass – *osteopenia* – is also seen in people with Type 1 diabetes.

FACT: Diabetes is associated with many joint and connective-tissue disorders.

SKIN CONDITIONS: some skin problems only appear in people with diabetes and can actually be a warning sign that complications will develop. This is the case because changes to the small blood vessels, and an increase in collagen – the protein found in cartilage and bone – are commonly seen in all complications.

DRY SKIN or EXCESSIVE SWEATING may be owing to your diabetes. People with diabetes may also find that the skin on their feet is dry because the feet don't sweat, but the face and upper body sweats profusely to compensate. People have also reported that eating foods like cheese cause them to sweat very heavily.

VITILIGO – loss of skin pigmentation – happens in people with Type 1 diabetes as part of the auto-immune process.

ACANTHOSIS NIGRICANS is a skin condition seen in Indian, Hispanic and black populations, causing velvety areas of dark pigmentation to form on the back of the neck and armpits. This condition can be improved with weight loss and the application of vitamin A and vitamin D creams.

NECROBIOSIS LIPOIDICA is a diabetes-related skin condition seen more frequently in women, where reddish-brown patches of skin form mostly on the shins and ankles, although it can also occur on the upper limbs and body and the face.

XANTHELASMA is another skin problem seen more often in people with diabetes, where small yellow fat deposits develop on the eyelids and other areas of skin. This can be an indicator that blood fats are high, so if these develop, go to your GP for blood tests to check fat levels. This condition can be associated with inflammation of the pancreas, which can lead to diabetes – if you don't already have it – because the organ swells and can't work properly. As with all complications of diabetes, treatment for xanthelasma involves tightening BG control.

> **FACT: Diabetes does not just affect your body physically – it can also affect your mental health.**

Case study: Judith

Judith Dixon was 33 when she had her first episode of severe depression. Her GP did not say that it would affect her diabetes in any way, but Judith found she could not meet the demands of trying to keep her BG under control. She had no interest in her usual social activities, so she gave up her keep-fit classes and cycling with her friends at weekends. She also lost interest in caring for herself, and stopped bothering about her hygiene or changing her clothes. She became so withdrawn, she rarely left the house. Judith couldn't explain why she felt the way she did but after two months, Judith's sister, Sandra, decided to make another appointment with the GP and, this time, Sandra went along to explain how Judith's depression was actually affecting her life. The GP prescribed some anti-depressants, but these had unpleasant side effects so Sandra took Judith to see her GP for a third time. She was prescribed a course of Cognitive Behavioural Therapy to help her recognise how her thoughts affected her feelings and behaviour. After sixteen sessions of this treatment, Judith's severe depression finally lifted.

DEPRESSION is three-times more likely to develop in people with diabetes than in people without the condition[19], although its cause is unknown. What is known is that a number of factors contribute towards the development of depression. For those with diabetes, one major added difficulty of depression is that it can lead to poor motivation for diabetes self-care. A person with diabetes suffering from depression might avoid administering their insulin injections or taking their glucose medication, as well as having regular blood tests and taking exercise.

Depression can also lead to higher BG levels because of hormonal and chemical changes in the body, and it can reoccur throughout a person's lifetime. Women tend to develop depression more often than men, and there are similar rates in people with Type 1 and Type 2 diabetes. Symptoms often go unnoticed for too long, so here are the things you should look out for[20]:

- Not being able to sleep.
- Feeling muddled.
- Having little or no energy.
- Getting easily upset.
- Feeling like you're not a worthwhile person.

19 Clark, M. (2004b), 'Identification and treatment of depression in people with diabetes', *Diabetes and Primary Care* 5(3), pp.124–7.
20 Ibid., pp.124–7.

- You may not feel like eating or you may over-eat to cheer yourself up.
- You don't feel like doing the normal activities you usually enjoy.
- You lose your sense of humour.
- You feel like you can't go on.

Depression can be treated with anti-depressant medication or with psycho-therapy, such as 'talking therapies'. Both work equally well, with 50–60 per cent[21] of people seeing an improvement in their symptoms after three months of treatment.

PREVENTION OF COMPLICATIONS

The best way to stop complications from developing, or stop them from getting worse if you already have them, is to aim to keep your BG tests between 5.0 and 7.0 mmol/L, meaning your HbA1c is as near the normal 6.0 per cent (42 mmol/L) as possible. This is easier said than done and can be practically impossible if you have dramatic swings in your BG. Regular BG tests enable you to see when you might need more or less insulin, or when your glucose medication is reducing your BG too much or not enough. It's important to work closely with your GP and/or diabetes consultant and nurse to get optimum control of your glucose levels. Preventing the onset of complications is the best possible motivation for good BG management.

Case study: Ellie

Ellie Watson developed Type 1 diabetes when she was eight and took her condition very seriously. When Ellie was 24, her mother,

21 Clark, M. (2004b), 'Identification and treatment of depression in people with diabetes', *Diabetes and Primary Care* 5(3), pp.124–7.

Jan – also with Type 1 – died from diabetes-related heart disease. Her mother had always been Ellie's motivation for looking after herself because, over the years, she also saw her mother go blind and have three toes amputated from her left foot because she didn't want to look after her diabetes.

Case study: Lucy

Lucy King had been taking insulin for a couple of years to treat her Type 2 diabetes. She never felt completely in control of her BG levels until she decided to keep a diary of her results. This helped her see patterns forming when she was higher or lower than she wanted. After a couple of weeks, Lucy realised she needed more insulin in the mornings and that she tended to dip down with much lower BG levels in the afternoon. She changed her insulin dosages accordingly and found her next HbA1c was 6.5 per cent (48 mmol/L).

FACT: **Having diabetes means lower-limb amputation is 15 to 70 times more likely.**

Your diabetes consultant and your GP will regularly want to see your feet so they can check for any diabetic changes. They will also check your urine for protein and the health of your eyes. As masters of our own diabetes, we're in the best position to know when something isn't quite right. It is also a very good idea if you check your own feet every day for cuts, blisters or sore patches, and report any problems or changes you notice in any part of your body as soon as possible to your GP. Foot care for people with diabetes is a priority and there are many chiropody and podiatry services specialising in foot care available that you can visit or that will even come to you if you have mobility problems.

FACT: **Foot problems in people with diabetes are the most preventable complications because changes like numbness or areas of hard skin can be detected quickly by you and can be speedily treated by your healthcare team.**

Exercising with foot problems

You may not think you have any problems with your feet, especially if you have no symptoms or pain, tingling, burning or numbness, or any areas of pressure and callouses that could become foot ulcers. Even if this is the case it's important to check your feet carefully every day for any changes. If you do have any diabetic changes, this is not an excuse to avoid exercising – you just have to make sure you exercise in a way that is appropriate and that won't make your foot problems worse. Remember – if you have any loss of sensation in your feet, you may not feel an injury:

- Make sure you change your footwear every five hours and don't wear tight trainers or shoes to exercise in as they will restrict the blood flow. A pair of cushioned trainers or a roomy pair – but not loose so they rub up and down – with gel insoles inserted makes a good choice of footwear.
- Make sure you don't wear socks with seams or holes that can rub part of your foot and cause a blister or a wound.
- If you do find an injury, blister, bruise or any other type of change when you remove your shoes/trainers, see a health professional as soon as possible to have it treated.

What else can I do to protect my feet?

- Make sure your shoes – and the seams on your socks – aren't rubbing and that your shoes aren't tight.
- Don't walk with bare feet.
- Shock-absorbing gel insoles can make a big difference by relieving pressure and foot pain.
- Make sure you don't have anything in your shoes, such as gravel from outside, before you put them on.
- Don't use hard skin removal 'sanding' machines with a spinning pumice stone; revolving toenail buffing/sanding devices; heated foot pads or vibrating foot massage machines.
- If you have problems finding shoes that fit, ask your GP, diabetes team or podiatrist for a referral to an *orthotist* at the hospital. This is a specially trained person who can make you made-to-measure shoes that will fit you perfectly so they won't rub and cause problems.
- Diabetes and smoking don't mix. Smoking clogs up blood vessels and reduces blood flow, increasing the risk of amputation.
- Wash and moisturise your feet daily. Do not use hot water and dry thoroughly before adding the cream – this is a must if the skin on your feet is very dry.
- If you do notice areas of pressure on your feet, stop wearing shoes that cause pressure.
- If you develop an area of skin on your foot that becomes infected – red around the edges, hot to the touch and 'squishy', or if pus has formed – inform your GP as soon as possible, raise the foot and rest it. Don't be tempted to walk on it!

Case study: Me!

I once knelt down to paint a skirting board and felt one of my toes go crack with the pressure of taking my weight in this position. I didn't feel any pain but found, after having it investigated, that I had broken my toe. So, be careful of putting any extra pressure on your toe joints by crouching down or stretching upwards on tip-toe.

THE EFFECTS OF CERTAIN MEDICATIONS AND OTHER HEALTH CONDITIONS ON YOUR BG

As I've mentioned before, people with diabetes often need more of certain vitamins as deficiencies can affect BG and hormone levels. The proper production of adrenal hormones, insulin – in Type 2 diabetes – and a substance known as *glucose tolerance factor* by the liver rely on good levels of vitamins C, B3, B5, B6, zinc and chromium. Because insulin is a hormone, it is affected by other levels of hormones, certain medications and other medical problems that you may also have.

MEDICATIONS AND NUTRITIONAL SUPPLEMENTS THAT INCREASE BG

Both prescribed medications and over-the-counter products can have a marked effect on your BG levels:

Statins – prescribed to reduce cholesterol levels – have been in the news because people who take these tablets have an increased risk of developing Type 2 diabetes as they raise BG levels, as well as increasing BG for those who already have Type 2. If you do take statins, it's advisable to carry on doing so because the risk of heart disease and stroke from having high cholesterol levels without statins is greater than an increase in BG when you take them.

Vitamin B3 – also known as nicotinic acid or *niacin* – reduces insulin production, affecting people with Type 2 diabetes by raising BG levels. This may be taken in a vitamin supplement or be prescribed by your GP to treat a high cholesterol level.

Thiazide tablets – *diuretics* or 'water tablets' – also have a tendency to increase BG levels because they reduce potassium levels in the body, meaning insulin is less able to lower BG levels. This is also the case for some tablets taken for high blood pressure[22] – *Atenolol, Bisoprolol, Minoxidil, Nifedipine* and *Amlodipine* – that alter the way the body processes glucose.

Some *corticosteroid* tablets prescribed for inflammatory conditions, and even some steroid creams used to treat and manage skin conditions like eczema, can increase BG levels. Some medications taken to prevent organ rejection following transplant, such as *Prednisone*, increase BG levels because they destroy the insulin-producing cells of the pancreas, meaning more insulin is needed for people with Type 2 diabetes.

Drug treatments for *psychosis* – severe mental disorder where thoughts and emotions are impaired – such[23] as *Chlorpromazine, Promazine, Fluphenazine* and *Tripfluoperazine* also reduce insulin production, meaning that BG levels are increased.

MEDICATIONS AND NUTRITIONAL SUPPLEMENTS THAT CAN DECREASE BG

Certain medications can reduce BG levels, as can some corticosteroids – always check the leaflet that comes with your prescription or over-the-counter medications. This is also the case for recreational drugs, like heroin, and sleeping pills, like barbiturates.

Alpha-blockers, such as *Doxazosin* derivatives that are used to treat high blood pressure, also have the effect of lowering BG, as do *fibric acid* derivatives used

---

22 https://insulinnation.com/non-diabetes-drugs-and-supplements-that-affect-glucose-levels

23 Ibid.

to treat fat disorders[24]. Fish oil supplements and aspirin taken at the same time can cause hypoglycaemia. Aspirin stops the absorption of glucose in the small intestine and Omega-3 fish oils have the same effect, meaning that frequent low BG levels can result. Aspirin also increases the effect of some BG-lowering medications taken to treat Type 2 diabetes.

Evening primrose oil interferes with the way BG-lowering medication – tablets or insulin – works with the effect that it further reduces BG levels.

FACT: A nutritional supplement that can improve eye health by reducing cell damage at the back of the eye is a combination of lutein and zeaxanthin. 20mg once a day can make vision sharper, reduce the prominence of eye 'floaters' and improve night vision.

MEDICAL CONDITIONS THAT ARE ASSOCIATED WITH HIGH BG LEVELS

Other than diabetes itself, there are several chronic (long-term) medical conditions that increase levels of BG:

Coeliac disease is an auto-immune condition triggered by an intolerance to gluten – a protein found in cereal grains, such as wheat – causing inflammation of the small bowel in the intestines. A gluten-free diet enables people with the disease to live perfectly healthily and, because gluten-free foods tend to have fewer carbohydrates, you will need less insulin.

There are several auto-immune conditions affecting the thyroid gland: *hypothyroidism* – an under-active thyroid gland; Graves' disease – an enlarged and *over-active thyroid gland*; and *Hashimoto's thyroiditis* – a condition causing

---

24 https://insulinnation.com/non-diabetes-drugs-and-supplements-that-affect-glucose-levels

the thyroid to produce less thyroid hormone. Too much thyroid hormone causes insulin to work for a shorter time and to be less effective. Increased levels of thyroid hormone cause the body to produce more glucose. The body's use of carbohydrate is also affected if there is not enough thyroid hormone, so the liver produces less glucose, reducing BG levels and increasing the risk of hypos. Although having an under-active thyroid usually results in lower BG levels, some people find instead that they have unexplained higher BG levels.

Case study: Wendy

Wendy Payne had Type 1 diabetes for 25 years when she was told she also had an under-active thyroid gland after routine blood tests. Wendy had been tired with no energy for a long time and her brain seemed very slow. Her GP started her on a low dose of thyroxine, but she didn't feel any different. Wendy had blood tests every three months and was told each time that the condition was getting worse. Her own BG tests were up and down without explanation and her diabetes consultant felt Wendy wasn't looking after herself properly. He warned that her mild sight problems would get more serious if she didn't do more to help herself. Wendy felt it wasn't her fault and read as much as she could about thyroid problems. She told her consultant that an under-active thyroid gland could cause high BG levels, but he disagreed with her that this was the problem. Eventually, Wendy's BG levels stabilised when she was put on a higher dose of thyroxine, proving Wendy was right.

Psoriasis is an auto-immune condition that affects the skin. It is now recognised that psoriasis is associated with a disruption in the production of insulin, increasing BG levels and leading to the later development of Type 2 diabetes. Obesity – defined as a body mass index of 30 and above – increases the risk of developing moderate to severe psoriasis. Psoriasis has also been linked to factors common in the development of Type 2 diabetes, such as the body not being able to manage glucose levels well. This means that psoriasis is more likely to develop when there is insulin resistance.

MEDICAL CONDITIONS THAT ARE ASSOCIATED WITH LOW BG LEVELS

As well as under-active thyroid conditions that may result in lower BG levels, other auto-immune conditions can reduce BG levels:

Addison's disease affects the adrenal glands that sit on top of the kidneys, and this condition can cause frequent and severe hypoglycaemia because it affects hormones that maintain the amount of glucose in the blood.

Insulinoma – a rare, non-cancerous tumour of the pancreas – secretes insulin and causes *unexplained hypoglycaemia*.

Pneumonia has the effect of reducing BG levels by making the body use up more glucose in response to fighting the infection.

Malaria can stimulate the body to produce more insulin.

Auto-immune syndrome[25] causes there to be a large amount of insulin in the bloodstream, despite BG already being low. Mostly, this insulin is inactive, but this situation can reverse.

Hereditary fructose disorder[26] causes low BG levels in children because their bodies can't use the sugars found in fruit.

Glycogen storage disease causes slow release of glucose by the liver and resulting hypoglycaemia. People with this problem are advised to eat slow-release

25 Marks, V. & Richmond, C. (2007), *Insulin Murders: True Life Cases.* (London: Royal Society of Medicine Press Limited).
26 Ibid.

carbohydrates like oats and bread so that their BG levels don't rise too quickly after a meal.

People with liver, kidney or glandular diseases might find they have low BG levels because the body uses glucose more quickly. Hypoglycaemia may also happen if a person suffers a long and severe lack of oxygen.[27]

27 Marks, V. & Richmond, C. (2007), *Insulin Murders: True Life Cases.* (London: Royal Society of Medicine Press Limited).

Chapter 9

DIABETES TRAINING COURSES

'It's not easy and it takes a lot of self-control, but it's definitely worth it.'

There are educational courses available for people with Type 1 or Type 2 diabetes to help them manage their condition as well as possible. Whatever type of diabetes you have, your GP, or practice or diabetes nurse will recommend an appropriate course and they will book you a place to attend at a venue that's local to you.

FACT: Most people with diabetes get only three hours a year with their GP, diabetes consultant and diabetes nurse – the rest of the time it's down to us to self-manage the condition.

MAKING FRIENDS WITH DAFNE IF YOU HAVE TYPE 1 DIABETES

For people with Type 1 diabetes who take insulin, the opportunity is there to live a virtually normal life eating what you like, when you like. This depends on knowing how much carbohydrate there is in the food you want to eat, how much insulin that carbohydrate requires, and how and when insulin will work to lower your BG so your levels stay within normal limits. The rate at which you digest food is also a factor. Autonomic nerve damage can slow down the rate of digestion, so that digestion takes many hours, making it difficult to match insulin needs – leading to hypos, then high BG levels once the insulin has worked but food is now available, raising BG levels.

DAFNE – what does this mean?

DAFNE stands for Dose Adjustment For Normal Eating. DAFNE is an educational course for people with Type 1 diabetes to give them the skills they need to administer the right amount of insulin for the amount of carbohydrate they choose to eat. Carbohydrate counting used to be a method emphasised by health professionals to control intake. This way of thinking then fell out of favour, but it's now back again with the new approach that you can count carbohydrates and have appropriate insulin to allow freedom in your lifestyle and food choices.

How long does the DAFNE course last?

The DAFNE course lasts for five days. There is a one-day follow-up after eight weeks to allow you to discuss your experiences and any problems you may have had.

How many people will be on the course with me?

The course is designed to involve a small group of six people with Type 1 diabetes. You can participate in discussions and share your experiences with the group and/or speak to the DAFNE trainer in private.

Is it worth me going, as I can already alter my insulin?

Although you may already be altering your insulin depending on carbohydrates eaten, the DAFNE course also offers vital information, education and support that really can help you to improve your diabetes control.

Can I go on a DAFNE course if I have Type 2 diabetes?

Even if you use insulin to treat your Type 2 diabetes, the DAFNE course is designed for people[1] with Type 1, which is a different form of

---

1   What is DAFNE? (2017) www.dafne.uk.com/What_is_DAFNE_-I293.html

diabetes and requires different management techniques to Type 2 diabetes. For these reasons, the DAFNE course is not offered to people with Type 2 diabetes.

Because people with Type 1 diabetes don't tend to be overweight, the aim of DAFNE is to be able to eat normally by calculating carbohydrate and necessary insulin dosages to keep BG levels normal. People with Type 2 diabetes taking insulin do so because their BG levels are not controlled as well by glucose-reducing medication. The aim for people with Type 2 diabetes is to control their BG levels by losing weight and cutting down on carbohydrates.

Will going on this course make a big change in my life?

One of the aims of the course is to help people accommodate diabetes into their lifestyle more easily so that they control their diabetes, rather than it controlling them. This means that making your insulin dosages appropriate for what you eat will be made as simple as possible, so you don't have to make huge changes to the way you do things at the moment.

What will I learn on the course?

The course covers all aspects of food and taking insulin[2]:

- How to count carbohydrate portions.
- How to set a background insulin dose – insulin that works all the time to keep your BG within normal range.
- How to take bolus insulin dosages – the insulin you give for meals, or when you have to bring down a high BG.
- How to correct BG levels when they are too high or too low.
- Managing BG levels and exercise.

2   What is DAFNE? (2017) www.dafne.uk.com/What_is_DAFNE_-I293.html

Case study: Justin

Justin Moore was 26 and had been struggling with his Type 1 diabetes for almost ten years. He checked his BG eight times a day and gave himself insulin if he was high, but he didn't know how much insulin he should be taking, so he usually ended up hypo a few hours later. He also usually had a hypo if he tried to take any exercise. Eventually Justin's diabetes consultant referred him for the DAFNE course when he realised that Justin's lifestyle was ruled by his diabetes. After attending the course, he felt he had a good understanding of how his diabetes affected him, what his BG results actually meant and how to act on them, and when his insulin was working. Justin was given step-by-step practical solutions to BG problems and five months later, his BG control was excellent – he knows exactly what he's doing with carbs and insulin rather than guessing.

FACT: Not every diabetes centre offers the DAFNE course because the course needs specially trained educators. If DAFNE is not available in your area, you can sign up to do an online version of the course at: www.dafne. uk.com

IF YOU HAVE TYPE 2

As we saw earlier, there are lifestyle changes we can all make to help reduce BG levels and the risk of developing serious complications:

- Increasing your amount of physical activity each day.
- Choosing healthy foods over high-fat, high-calorie alternatives.

- Understanding prescribed medications – what they're for, when to take them and how much.
- Working with the health professionals who look after you.

Even if you find adapting to these lifestyle changes difficult, remember that you don't have to face them on your own. Encourage your family and friends to eat healthily with you (it's good for everyone), and find someone to exercise with so that the process feels sociable and connected, rather than lonely.

FACT: As with any major change, start gradually. If you try to make all the changes at once, you will find the process overwhelming and you'll be more likely to give up.

Start by doing little things that will make a big difference, like swapping sugary drinks for diet or sugar-free ones; reducing or adding no sugar to the hot drinks and meals you make at home; and reducing the quantity of sweet snacks, like biscuits, cake and chocolate, that you eat each day. Like any habit, this new way of managing your diet will take time to become something you do without even thinking about it.

FACT: It takes three weeks to break a bad habit such as eating a daily bar of chocolate. Establishing the new one – such as eating a piece of fruit every day – takes three months.

In the same way as making different food choices, you could make changes to the amount of physical activity you do – if you are able to – by making the choice to walk rather than drive short distances; by walking for longer; and climbing stairs rather than using an escalator or lift. Think about what are achievable goals for you.

> **FACT:** Type 2 diabetes is a health condition that you can do something about if you make changes to your lifestyle.

GETTING TO KNOW DESMOND IF YOU HAVE TYPE 2 DIABETES[3]

DESMOND stands for Diabetes Education and Self-Management for Ongoing and Newly Diagnosed. Your GP or practice nurse will recommend this course, which is run by experts in Type 2 diabetes – nurses, dieticians and diabetes educators. It's designed to help you understand and get to grips with your diagnosis, providing you with useful information about how to manage your diabetes. At the DESMOND course, you will meet other people who have also just recently been diagnosed with Type 2 diabetes and the course leaders will encourage you to discuss any worries you have about looking after yourself.

Case study: Doreen

Doreen Brown was in her early 70s when her GP told her that she had Type 2 diabetes. Doreen was very shocked as she had not felt unwell. She felt it was silly to start worrying about changing what she ate and doing more exercise. Doreen was invited to attend the DESMOND course and she went along, expecting it to be of little interest to her. She was surprised to find a small, friendly group of people attending the course who had the same feelings and worries as her own, and they shared ideas and offered support. She found out how to make sensible food choices and why it was important to

---

3 'Getting to Grips with Type 2 Diabetes' (2010). See www.desmond-project.co.uk.

make an effort to improve her health. She began to change the portion sizes of her meals, eating half as many potatoes every day and cutting out biscuits. She still made her own cakes, but Doreen cut the sugar in the recipe by two-thirds. When Doreen had another diabetes check three months later at her GP surgery, she was told that her condition was so much improved, her BG was now normal.

It's a good idea to write down anything you want to ask. Because you are going into a new situation and you have many things on your mind, you may forget what you wanted to say. The course will focus mainly on food groups and how these affect your BG. Changes in diet are always of more benefit when you also make changes to improve your physical activity levels.

ASSESSING YOUR PHYSICAL ACTIVITY

You might think you are fairly active already because, for example, you walk your dog every day or make a daily trip to the shops on foot. Being physically active is unique to each individual – if you are middle aged and physically active in your job, your needs are quite different to someone who is older and has arthritis and can't move around very easily. Whatever your starting point, aim to increase the **amount** of activity you do each day if you can. This doesn't mean that you have to join a gym or start jogging around the park every morning; it can be bending and flexing your legs at the knees or lifting your arms up and down while you are sitting watching television.

FACT: **Every movement burns glucose. When you have diabetes, strengthening your muscles is very important in order to maintain good mobility.**

Health practitioners recommend certain levels of physical activity, just as they do our nutritional intake. Recommendations are for 30 minutes of moderately intensive activity – meaning activity that makes you feel warmer and increases your breathing and heart rate a little – at least five times a week. However, health problems in some people will make this really tricky to achieve. It's important to know, in that case, that the recommended activity doesn't have to be 30 continuous minutes – you can break it up into chunks. Of course, if you have asthma, you may get breathless climbing stairs or bending to use a dustpan and brush. The point is that as long as you are increasing the amount of physical activity you do, your diabetes management will benefit.

FACT: Asthma inhalers – Ventolin, also known as Salbutamol – stimulate the pancreas to produce insulin.

Exercise is basically movement and it does not have to be a sporting activity that you specifically make time to do. How much glucose you burn off depends on the length of time you do the activity and how much movement is involved. Housework involves some good glucose-burning activities and, while I can't tell you how many BG points you'll burn off if you do them, I can tell you the calories you will burn. A calorie is a measurement of heat – you get hot when you are physically active, because you are burning calories as well as glucose. If the activity burns a lot of calories quickly, it also burns a lot of glucose. The following table[4] shows how long you have to do various housework activities to burn 100 calories, although this is only an average and is also dependent on your gender, weight and fitness levels:

---

4   Physical activity and calories. In 'Getting to Grips with Type 2 Diabetes' (2010). See www.desmond-project.co.uk.

Household activity	Time to burn 100 calories
Digging the garden	12 minutes
Shovelling snow	15 minutes
Weeding the garden	18 minutes
Painting the house	18 minutes
Washing the car	20 minutes
Mowing the lawn	20 minutes
Mopping the floor	20 minutes
Vacuuming	22 minutes
Raking leaves	23 minutes
Playing with your children/carrying a child	24 minutes
Cleaning the house	25 minutes
Shopping	25 minutes
Walking a dog	26 minutes
Pushing a pram	35 minutes
Ironing	50 minutes
Washing dishes	50 minutes

The 'Preparing for DESMOND' pamphlet suggests that you assess how active you are by answering true or false to the following questions[5]:

- I do some activity in my home on most days – housework, gardening, and so on.
- I try to be moderately active for 30 minutes most days.
- I always walk instead of driving, if I can.
- I'm very active as part of my job/daily routine.

You may have found you were less active than you thought. Use this list to help you increase your activity levels each day.

5   'Preparing for DESMOND' (2010). See www.desmond-project.org.uk.

THINKING ABOUT YOUR FOOD CHOICES

We've already talked about calories and controlling your weight, but as with physical activity, you may not realise what you're actually eating until you write it down. Keep a food diary before you go on your DESMOND course. Be honest as you don't have to share it with anyone else. This method really does help you see where your calories are coming from – a couple of biscuits with every cup of tea, for example, might mean an extra 300 calories a day that you don't really notice you're eating because they're not main meals. Just be aware of what you're eating and why – we often eat through boredom or because we want to cheer ourselves up. Add how you feel to your diary entry. This is a good way of controlling your food choices a little better because you become aware of eating when you're not hungry.

Looking at what you eat will enable the DESMOND sessions to help you. The following are some of the questions the course will raise[6]:

- Do you eat the same sorts of foods each day?
- What do you usually have for breakfast?
- What do you normally have for lunch?
- What are you eating for your main meal each day?
- What snack(s) do you eat?

Look at the answers you've given and go back to when we looked at the fat and calorie contents of foods. What changes do you think you could make to your diet to improve your diabetes control? You will be able to talk about making these changes on the DESMOND course.

BEING AWARE OF YOUR MOODS

As you've already seen, BG control is hugely affected by your emotions and how you feel – feeling unhappy increases BG, while, if you have a good day,

6 'Preparing for DESMOND' (2010). See www.desmond-project.org.uk.

your BG may be well controlled. This is another aspect of the DESMOND course[7] that you'll be able to discuss to get more support for living with and managing your diabetes. It's common to find it hard to accept the diagnosis of diabetes and you may want to also write your moods in your food and activity diary as they are related – such as eating for comfort when feeling sad and only doing what's absolutely necessary in terms of physical activity – gardening or decorating the house will not be at the top of your list if you feel fed up. Make a note of things like:

- When something has really bothered you.
- If you feel miserable, even if your friends and family try to cheer you up.
- If you feel your self-esteem is really low – 'I'm stupid'; 'I'm not as good as she is'; and so on.
- When your mind wanders and you dwell on negative thoughts.
- If you feel depressed.
- If you have little interest in food and lose your appetite.
- When everything seems too much trouble.
- If you can't sleep and find yourself worrying.
- If you feel very emotional.
- If you feel unhappy, isolated and lonely.
- When you have no energy to do anything.
- When you feel happy and you think your life is going well.

The answers you give can show you how well you are coping with your diagnosis and living with your diabetes. If you feel sad and low much of the time, go and see your doctor who will be able to help and provide support. Your notes on food, activity and mood will not only help you recognise patterns of behaviour in your life, they are also points to discuss with the DESMOND course trainers.

---

7   'What about my feelings?' In: 'Preparing for DESMOND' (2010). See www.desmond-project.org.uk.

Chapter 10

Reversing Type 2 Diabetes

'There are barriers to health, but the barrier should not be you.'

Type 2 diabetes is thought to occur in 90 per cent of cases because the person eats a high-fat, high-carbohydrate diet and takes little or no exercise. Some people with Type 2 have actually been on the receiving end of stigma where others have blamed them, saying that they have brought this on themselves. Some with Type 2 have stated that they feel blamed by health professionals and misunderstood by those with Type 1 diabetes, which isn't related to lifestyle.

Case study: Abdul

Abdul Yusef was once at a diabetes clinic where a woman started shouting at him, saying there was nothing she could do about her Type 1 diabetes, whereas his was self-inflicted from eating too much and not exercising, and that he was lucky because all he had to do was lose weight to get rid of his Type 2.

Case study: Amanda

Amanda Farah had been told several times by nurses, doctors and dieticians that her Type 2 diabetes was all in her own hands, that she had made herself like that because she had no self-control or motivation to exercise, and that she didn't care about her body or what she ate.

Can changing what i eat and how i exercise actually reverse Type 2 diabetes?

In recent years the number of people developing Type 2 diabetes in the UK has soared by 65 per cent so that 3.5 million are now living with the condition. This current epidemic – for most people, but not all – is caused by physical inactivity and obesity. The problem is now so great that health professionals in the UK cannot keep up with the number of new diagnoses. As we have just seen, the aim of the DESMOND course is to help people with Type 2 diabetes manage their condition as well as they can. Once you have the information, education and support provided by the DESMOND course, you are equipped to improve your BG control.

FACT: Dieting alone will not reverse your Type 2. Reversal is possible only with a complete change involving healthy eating and regular exercise.

How low are low-carbohydrate and low-fat diets?

Research shows[1] that people with Type 2 diabetes who adopted a low-carbohydrate diet of less than 20g carbohydrate – the equivalent of a small apple – a day for six months, but without any calorie restrictions for protein and fat, achieved reduced BG levels and improved HbA1c results. Because carbohydrates convert to glucose in the body, low-carbohydrate diets help prevent any rise in blood glucose levels. Cutting out or strictly reducing the amount of carbohydrate you eat reduces or avoids the need to take glucose-reducing medication. Lifestyle change can reverse Type 2 diabetes if you are very motivated to achieve this goal, but you must talk to your diabetes

---

1   Holford, P. (2011), *Say No to Diabetes: 10 Secrets to Preventing and Reversing Diabetes.* (London: Piatkus).

consultant before cutting down on carbohydrates as your diabetes medication will need to be altered.

Case study: Molly

Molly Khan weighed 95kg and was told she had Type 2 diabetes. She read about a lifestyle-change programme in the USA involving a low-calorie, low-fat diet with moderate exercise each day. Health professionals supervised the programme and the people taking part successfully lost weight and reversed their diabetes after following the programme for four months. The participants were told that they needed to continue to lose weight until they reached a normal BMI calculation. Once they had reversed their diabetes and achieved a normal body weight, they continued a healthy eating and exercise plan as part of their new lifestyle. A couple of people went back to their old ways of eating high-fat, high-carbohydrate foods and doing little or no exercise and their diabetes returned. Molly realised she needed to make a complete change to her lifestyle, consulted her GP and, after six months of determined effort, she had lost 21kg and her Type 2 diabetes was gone. Molly has stuck to her new lifestyle plan and is determined to never have Type 2 diabetes again.

FACT: Eating a low-carbohydrate diet is not the same as a low-calorie diet. Low-carbohydrate diets allow a normal amount of fat, meaning they are not low-calorie.

You may be advised to lose weight quickly if you require surgery – such as joint replacement – which may mean a very low-calorie diet of less than 800 calories a day. You will be allowed to stay on such a calorie-restricted diet for only twelve weeks because vitamin and mineral deficiency can develop – your weight loss and general health will be supervised during this time. If you have chronic complications such as reduced liver or kidney function, cardiac impairment, disordered eating or psychological health problems, a restricted diet may not be suitable for you.

WEIGHT-LOSS SURGERY

Weight-loss surgery, such as fitting a gastric band, has been suggested as the way to effectively tackle Type 2 diabetes in the population because it costs so much to treat the condition. Surgery may be the best option for someone who is *morbidly obese* – defined as a Body Mass Index of 45 and above – as low-carbohydrate and low-calorie diets may not be suitable. Keeping motivation high for losing weight is a major problem for people with Type 2 diabetes, but finding out why people overeat can be cheaper for the NHS than surgery.

Case study: Suzanne

Suzanne Ryan had always had a weight problem and, when she was 42, she developed Type 2 diabetes. With the help of a dietician and a clinical psychologist at the hospital, she discovered that she often ate for comfort. It was a vicious circle: she was then unhappy because she was fat. Suzanne realised she was often just eating for the sake of it and not because she was hungry. By changing her way of thinking, Suzanne managed to lose 19kg and now her BG control is normal. Her diabetes consultant has said that if she keeps the weight off, she will continue to have normal BG readings – Suzanne no longer needs to take diabetes medication.

Case study: Dave

Dave Norris developed Type 2 diabetes when he was 35 because he viewed food as a comfort – although it was only once he'd seen a counsellor for three months that he realised his eating was related to the fact that he had spent lots of time in care homes as a child and had been adopted. After counselling, every time Dave thought about eating junk food, he reminded himself of what he'd discussed with his counsellor. His diabetes control is now much improved and his consultant is hoping Dave can come off Metformin completely in the near future.

FACT: **Excess body fat interferes with how insulin works in body cells, causing insulin resistance and raised BG levels. Weight loss means that an amount of fat is removed from the body, so insulin is able to work normally, improving BG control.**

So, an improved diet and regular cardiovascular exercise holds the promise of reversing Type 2 diabetes without the potentially dangerous side effects of surgery. But this lifestyle change must be tailored to your specific needs by appropriately trained health professionals providing you with ongoing assistance and encouragement. As with weight-loss surgery, diet and exercise is not a quick-fix solution, and the changes you make must become permanent. This means you must be very motivated to succeed so that you keep going.

Obesity is a significant risk factor for the development of many health conditions including heart disease; Type 2 diabetes; high blood pressure (*hypertension*); abnormal blood fats, such as high cholesterol; stroke; fatty deposits in the arteries (*atherosclerosis*); and some types of cancer. Obesity is not only a risk factor for serious physical disease; it also leads to psychological conditions such as depression, disordered eating and a reduced quality of life, with complications increasing with the duration of obesity.

FACT: More than a quarter of UK adults are now classed as obese and a further 42 per cent of men and 33 per cent of women are overweight.

It is thought that 1.4 million morbidly obese people – with a BMI above 35 – could benefit from weight-loss surgery, potentially reversing 40,000 cases of Type 2 diabetes and 5,000 cases of heart disease[2]. In 2016 the NHS stated that it spends £17 billion on obesity-related conditions every year. A weight loss of 5–10 per cent hugely improves conditions like Type 2 diabetes and heart disease that are made worse by excess body fat. People who are morbidly obese can't achieve weight loss with diet and exercise alone, so they are considered for surgery. The need to lose weight and improve the effects of Type 2 diabetes and heart disease outweighs the risks that come with a weight-loss operation.

FACT: Having a gastric band fitted to drastically reduce the size of the stomach is not an easy option and it is not a quick fix. Anyone who has this surgery must also make significant changes to their diet and exercise lifestyle in order for the surgery to be successful.

---

2   Owen-Smith, A. (2016), 'Experience of accessing obesity surgery on the NHS', *Journal of Public Medicine*. See https://academic.oup.com/jpubhealth/article/ 39/1/163/3065701

Case study: Dee

Dee Vanson-Luis had a gastric band fitted to reduce the size of her stomach, but she didn't utilise the support to motivate her to make it work. She stuck to the diet after her surgery, eating very small meals for about a month. Then she started to cheat – having ice cream and full-fat coffees – so she actually regained the 4.5kg she'd lost after having the gastric band fitted, plus a bit more. Dee had to eventually confess to her doctor what she'd been doing and he threatened to remove the band if she wasn't going to use it properly. She felt so guilty and ashamed, it forced her to take control.

How weight-loss surgery works

There are two basic types of weight-loss surgery: *restrictive surgery* and *reduced absorption* with restrictive surgery[3]:

- Restrictive surgery physically makes the size of the stomach much smaller (about 80 per cent smaller) to slow down digestion to give a feeling of fullness for longer with less food.
- Reduced absorption with restrictive surgery involves physically removing a portion of the digestive tract to restrict the number of calories that the body can absorb.

The insertion of an adjustable gastric band – also known as lap-band surgery – is one example of restrictive surgery. This involves placing a synthetic band around the upper portion of the stomach to form a small pouch to significantly reduce the amount of food and calories that you can eat. The surgeon can inflate or deflate the band through a port beneath the skin on the abdomen in order to change the size of the stomach. The band can be removed

3   Keidar, A. (2011), 'Bariatric surgery for Type 2 diabetes reversal: the risks', *Diabetes Care* 34(2), S361–S367.

at any time. Other procedures create a 'sleeve' where a small portion of the stomach is sectioned off so that it needs less food to become full, and surgery can reduce the size of the stomach and intestine to limit the food and calories your body absorbs.

FACT: Severe vitamin deficiency can happen after having weight-loss surgery.

Reversing Type 2 diabetes with surgery

The reversal of Type 2 diabetes with surgery was first seen more than ten years ago, although certain methods are better than others. These methods have been successful in returning BG, insulin production and HbA1c to normal in 80–100 per cent of morbidly obese people with Type 2 diabetes. Research shows that normal BG and insulin levels happen within days after surgery, despite the fact that there's been little or no weight loss[4]. This means that, despite the fact there is no significant weight loss, insulin is still able to work much better. It is possible that these results are owing to the combination of smaller meals, reduced absorption of nutrients, and a change in the gastrointestinal – GI – tract affecting how the body uses glucose.

FACT: Because of the ability of weight-loss surgery to reverse Type 2 diabetes, this will help develop new treatments for both Type 2 and obesity in the future.

---

4   Keidar, A. (2011), 'Bariatric surgery for Type 2 diabetes reversal: the risks', *Diabetes Care* 34(2), S361–S367.

Research shows that the successful reversal of Type 2 diabetes with surgery means[5]:

- Being able to stop taking BG-lowering medication.
- Normal BG levels in up to 86.6 per cent of people.
- 80 per cent of people become diabetes-free.
- Normal levels of insulin.
- An average weight loss of 44kg.

FACT: **People who have had Type 2 for less than five years and who have controlled their condition with diet achieve the best BG control after weight-loss surgery.**

Possible complications following weight-loss surgery

Weight-loss surgery is associated with some complications depending on the type of procedure. The simpler restrictive procedures like gastric banding rarely affect the function of the bowel, so there's less risk of vitamin deficiency unless you have repeated sickness. Stomach acid can erode the synthetic band, causing abdominal pain and reduced weight loss. Sometimes the consultant may over-fill the band so that it slips down the stomach, making a bigger pouch for food, meaning there is no weight loss – or there may even be weight gain.

Surgery designed to reduce the absorption of nutrients is a serious procedure. There may be problems in the first few months after surgery such as[6]:

- Poor wound healing – a particular difficulty in people with diabetes.
- Incision hernias – pushing part of the digestive tract out of its

---

5 Keidar, A. (2011), 'Bariatric surgery for Type 2 diabetes reversal: the risks', *Diabetes Care* 34(2), S361–S367.
6 Ibid., S361–S367.

normal position – after bypass and re-joining parts of the small bowel to reduce the absorption of nutrients.

- Obstruction of the small bowel in 2.1 per cent of cases.
- Narrowing of the small bowel in 0.7 per cent of surgeries.
- Gastrointestinal bleeding in 0.6 per cent of surgeries.
- Leakage of the contents of the small bowel at the incision site in 1.2 per cent of cases.
- Artery blockage by a blood clot – pulmonary embolus – in 1.0 per cent of surgeries.
- Pneumonia in 0.1–0.3 per cent of surgeries.

There are other longer-term complications following gastrointestinal surgery such as:

- Lack of protein absorption causing swelling of the lower limbs and a feeling of weakness.
- Calcium, iron and vitamin deficiencies. (Small portion sizes must provide good nutrient quantities, plus there will be a need for vitamin supplementation.)
- Prolonged vomiting, the growth of scar tissue causing narrowing and/ or poor intestinal absorption of nutrients.

FACT: Research shows a 92-per-cent reduction in deaths from Type 2 diabetes because of weight-loss surgery.

Case study: Teresa

Teresa Bull had a gastric band fitted and was told, to her delight, that she no longer had Type 2 diabetes. She frequently had heart-burn and had been vomiting regularly as a complication of her surgery and six months later, Teresa developed nerve and circulatory problems owing to a lack of vitamin B1. She had mild peripheral neuropathy affecting the nerves in her feet because of high BG levels when she had diabetes, but it became much worse after her weight-loss surgery. Blood tests showed severe vitamin deficiencies, including iron, vitamin D and calcium, making her feel tired and weak, with muscle pain. Teresa also found she was often constipated because much less food was passing through, and she developed gallstones. She was prescribed high dosages of vitamins to correct her deficiencies and laxatives to help her constipation. Despite all the side effects she experienced, Teresa feels it was worth having the surgery because she has lost 13.5kg in weight and no longer takes BG-lowering medication.

The UK's Department of Health agrees that weight-loss surgery to reverse Type 2 is an excellent way to prevent diabetic complications in people recently diagnosed. This is because it is better to prevent complications than to have the cost of needing to treat them. Tighter or near-normal BG results can have a positive effect on the prevalence of complications, but fundamentally the damage is done and irreversible.

Case study: Patty

Patty Deane paid to have weight-loss surgery two years ago. She used to take insulin for her Type 2 diabetes and, almost as soon as she'd had the operation, she didn't have to inject anymore, even though she hadn't actually lost much weight. Unfortunately, she'd already developed eye and nerve complications that have not improved or gone away, despite the fact Patty's BG is now normal and so is her HbA1c.

FACT: Having a BMI of 35 and above reduces life-expectancy by ten years.

Case study: Dev

Dev Patel was advised to have surgery to lose weight and help his diabetes. It sounded like a great idea. His consultant explained the risks of surgery (including fatality), but they didn't seem real when he was sitting in the consultant's office. Dev just wanted to lose weight and feel better. He had problems after the operation and was very ill, needing a long stay in hospital. Although he doesn't regret surgery, he wishes he'd fully accepted how different his relationship with food would be afterwards. He misses eating as he previously did, despite having lost 32kg and improving his BG.

How much weight would I lose?

There is an average 47.5-per-cent loss in bodyweight for people who have a gastric band fitted and 61.6 per cent of total bodyweight for those who undergo gastric bypass surgery. Weight loss tends to stabilise at around two years following surgery, and there can even be some weight gain by the third year. Perhaps more important than weight loss is the significant reversal of various weight-related health conditions. *Metabolic syndrome* – a collection of conditions that accompany Type 2 diabetes – can also be reversed with weight-loss surgery so that an early death, with its associated cardiac risk factors, is avoidable.

How will I adjust to eating much less?

Weight-loss surgery is an extremely successful way to treat obesity and reverse Type 2 diabetes to delay and stabilise the chronic and life-threatening complications of the disease. But what about the effect on mental health when the person has to live a life of forced change, which they may not be fully prepared for, despite psychological counselling? A lot has been written about the physical complications of weight-loss surgery, but much less about the psychological effects. Before and after surgery, it is known that[7]:

- Morbidly obese people experience mood disorders, anxiety and low self-esteem and are five times more likely to have suffered from major depression in the previous five years when compared with average-weight individuals.

- Depression is common among morbidly obese individuals. One major factor is body dissatisfaction, especially for women (it's thought owing to images of 'perfection' in the media).

- There is a stigma attached to obesity, leading to prejudice and discrimination, which causes or worsens depression.

- Yo-yo dieting exacerbates symptoms of depression, such as hopelessness and low self-esteem, where weight-loss attempts fail.

- 20–30 per cent of people report symptoms of depression relating to body image and low self-esteem at the time of their weight-loss surgery, with 50 per cent saying they have a life-long history of depression – these factors probably contribute to any decision to go ahead with the operation in the first place.

Psychological health is closely associated with further weight gain in obese individuals and people having weight-loss surgery are more likely to suffer psychological distress compared with obese patients who don't have surgery. The trigger for some people to seek out this type of surgery – rather than a doctor advising it – is usually a traumatic or distressing event, such as the death of a loved one. Poor psychological health is also associated with Type 2 diabetes and obesity. As we have already seen, the impact of living with multiple health problems such as diabetes-related heart disease, blindness,

7   Abiles V, et al. (2010), 'Psychological characteristics of morbidly obese candidates for bariatric surgery', *Obesity Surgery* 20(2), pp.161–7.

kidney disease, and/or nerve pain takes a massive toll on the individual physically and mentally.

Who can have weight-loss surgery?

To be eligible for this type of procedure, you must have been unable to lose weight with diet and exercise and have a BMI of above 35 if you have Type 2 diabetes[8]. Because weight-loss surgery enforces extreme dietary change it is expected that the person will adopt lifestyle change regarding their eating and exercise habits. The selection of suitable candidates for weight-loss surgery involves an in-depth assessment of medical, psychological and social issues and measures are taken to assess the potential psychological impact of surgery. It is known that after surgery there is:

- An improvement in depressive symptoms for 2–4 years, higher self-esteem, health-related quality of life, and a more positive body image.
- With good adaptation to behaviour change, a substantial decrease in depression and anxiety in the year following the procedure, compared to obese individuals who underwent diet and exercise counselling.
- Particular improvement in the symptoms of depression and anxiety.

Despite the stunning success rate of weight-loss surgery in reversing obesity-related health conditions and improving overall physical and mental health, there is still a minority of people who don't feel that weight-loss surgery has been a positive experience. Some find they don't have any long-term health gains or benefit following weight-loss surgery. This may be because these people had unrealistic expectations of a dramatic change in their life following their surgery, setting themselves up for disappointment. It means that even if such people lose a large amount of weight, appearing

---

8   National Institute for Health and Care Excellence (NICE) (2014b), Press release: 'NICE updates weight-loss surgery criteria for people with Type 2 diabetes'. See nice.org.uk/cg190.

to fall short of their own expectations has a negative effect on their mental health.

Case study: Laura

Laura Swain was 33 when she paid to have weight-loss surgery to reverse her Type 2 diabetes. She felt she had been stupid in expecting life to be different after she went through the surgery and lost weight. Laura had imagined that she'd be more popular, that she'd be invited out and be the life and soul of the party. In reality, her life hasn't changed at all – it's exactly the same except that she's thinner. She still has the same problems in her private life. While she admits she has more confidence now to move to another job or house to make a better life, Laura feels she was expecting too much from the surgery. Laura was blaming her weight for problems in her life but now realises that there are further issues she needs to tackle.

Support for making surgery work

After weight-loss surgery it's important to receive support and regular contact with health professionals. It is known that after the first year, as clinic appointments in which health professionals offer encouragement become fewer, the symptoms of depression can increase because the person feels they are now on their own.

Will the surgery increase self-confidence?

The person's view of how they appear to others after weight-loss surgery influences their sense of self-confidence, attractiveness and body image. This is unique to each person and this, in turn, enhances the individual's personality. Because weight-loss surgery can change body shape dramatically it's associated with increased self-esteem, self-confidence and personality because of an improved body image and weight-loss satisfaction. However, because the skin stretches with stored body fat, it may not spring back again when weight is lost because this ability decreases as we get older. This may cause significant distress.

Case study: Joe

Joe Beresford was 28 when he lost 63.5kg having had a gastric band fitted, exercising for 30 minutes every day and cutting out sweet and fatty foods. After his dramatic weight loss, his Type 2 diabetes disappeared but his new 76kg shape had folds of skin hanging from his arms, legs and chest. He hadn't expected to have so much loose skin and he viewed this as ugly. Despite this, Joe was pleased with his overall appearance and he felt good about his body image. Joe has arranged to have a second operation to remove the skin on the underside of his arms and more surgery to have his legs done, a tummy tuck and a bottom lift. He is prepared for the extensive scars everywhere but wishes he'd now got the body he dreamed of. He just wanted the fat to be gone when he woke up after the surgery.

Can children have weight-loss surgery?

There are now increasing cases of children who are developing Type 2 diabetes because they eat an unhealthy diet and do little or no exercise. Escalating rates of extreme obesity in children are being reported and with this alarming trend comes not only Type 2 diabetes, but also other 'adult' diseases such as *obstructive sleep apnoea* (where fat around the neck impairs breathing during sleep); fatty liver disease; and heart disease, with severely obese adolescents being at particular risk[9]. Obese children are also known to experience significant hostility from others; low self-esteem; body dissatisfaction; depressive

---

9   Kubik, J. F., et al. (2013), 'The impact of bariatric surgery on psychological health', *Journal of Obesity*. See http://dx,doi.org/10,1155/2013/837989.

symptoms; poor food choices; and harmful weight-control behaviours such as *anorexia* and/or *bulimia*. They also are less able to be sociable and make friends. The problems are worse in girls than boys.

FACT: Tackling the problem of childhood obesity involves the whole family understanding portion control. Reducing calories and increasing the amount of regular exercise will benefit the whole family.

Weight-loss surgery is considered for young people with life-threatening obesity, but only in extreme cases where the need outweighs the risk. Rather, doctors prefer that children try diet, exercise and weight-loss medication first. The success rate of weight-loss surgery in adolescents is similar to that in adults, with 40–60 per cent of excess weight lost in the first year and upwards of 75 per cent by the end of the second year[10].

Weight-loss surgery in young adults has the effect of improving high blood pressure; insulin resistance; Type 2 diabetes; and high levels of unhealthy blood fats. Psychologically, depression, anxiety and self-image are also improved following stomach-reducing procedures after as little as four months, and this improvement lasts for more than four years. This shows that mental health is strongly associated with weight control.

FACT: A weight-loss surgeon must feel that the need to improve the health of a young person is greater than the risk of having the surgery.

---

10 Hsia, D. S., Fallon, S. C., Brandt, M. L. (2012), 'Adolescent Bariatric Surgery', *Archives of Pediatric & Adolescent Medicine* 166(8), pp.757–66.

Chapter 11

What Diabetes Care Should I Receive?

'Going into hospital worries me because I can't be in control of my diabetes.'

Your Basic Rights

As a person with diabetes in the UK, you are entitled to receive a certain level of care – this will be different in countries such as the USA and Australia where healthcare is dependent on health insurance. Care in the UK is laid down by UK law so if you don't get the right treatment, it's possible to take the matter to court. You may not have previously even questioned diabetes care in your area or know what the correct sort of care is. There are certain rights that you should have as standard without having to ask, such as[1]:

- Getting most healthcare free of charge.
- Being able to have the GP you want, although they can refuse you. If you can't find a GP in your area, your Local Authority can help. You can also change your GP when you like without giving them notice.
- The right to see your medical records. This can be refused if it's felt that seeing them may cause you distress, or if a third party is mentioned in part of the records who has said they don't want the records to be seen.
- The right to refuse treatment, unless it's covered by the Mental Health Act, 1983.
- The right for your information to be confidential within the NHS as part of your treatment.

1 Diabetes UK (2000), *What Diabetes Care to Expect* (London: Diabetes UK).

- The right for any complaint you make against the NHS to be investigated using the NHS complaints procedure.
- Possible refund of travel costs to hospital, NHS prescription charges, NHS dental charges, and NHS sight tests, glasses and contact lenses, wigs and fabric supports. Your local Benefit Agency will have information about refunds.

FACT: **Make sure you know what you're entitled to so that your needs as a person with diabetes are met.**

So, now you know your rights to general healthcare, but what about your rights to specialist diabetes care? Recent reports in the news have highlighted patchy diabetes care across the country. To get the best out of the system you need to be prepared to work with health professionals so that you are **part** of your diabetes team. After all, **you** are the most important person in this team! Knowing as much as you can about your diabetes is the key to being able to discuss your condition and getting what you need to manage it properly.

FACT: **You can discuss the roles and responsibilities of your diabetes care team with your GP.**

WHO'S WHO? YOUR DIABETES CARE TEAM INCLUDES[2]:

- You
- Your diabetes consultant, also known as your diabetologist or endocrinologist.

2 Diabetes UK (2000), *What Diabetes Care to Expect.* (London: Diabetes UK).

- Your diabetes specialist nurse – DSN.
- Your General Practitioner – GP.
- Your Practice Nurse at your GP surgery.
- A dietician.
- An optometrist or ophthalmologist to care for your eyes.
- A podiatrist or chiropodist to care for your feet.
- A psychologist or diabetes-trained counsellor.
- Your pharmacist.

You may see some members of your diabetes team more often than others, especially when you are first diagnosed. As this is the time when everything is new and you are having to take in lots of information about your condition, your diabetes team should[3]:

- Provide you with a full medical examination.
- Decide on a plan of diabetes care with you.
- Introduce you to a diabetes specialist nurse who will explain the condition, your treatment and how to use diabetes self-care equipment such as a BG-testing monitor.
- Teach you how to manage your own diabetes.
- Arrange a meeting with a dietician so you can discuss what you eat and get advice on how to improve your diet to help your BG control.
- Explain the importance of a healthy diet and regular exercise.
- Explain how diabetes may affect your lifestyle in terms of issues such as work, driving a vehicle, travel and life insurance.
- Provide ongoing information and education about diabetes-related issues as necessary.
- Give you information about local diabetes support groups.

3   Diabetes UK (2000), *What Diabetes Care to Expect* (London: Diabetes UK).

> **FACT:** Once your diabetes is under control you will see your
> diabetes team at least once a year for an annual review,
> although you should be able to contact them for advice
> when you need it.

AFTER YOU HAVE MET YOUR DIABETES TEAM, THEY SHOULD PROVIDE YOU WITH[4]:

- Ongoing care based on a full knowledge of your needs and medical history.
- Periodic review to help you achieve your diabetes management goals.
- The opportunity to be involved in your diabetes-care decisions.
- Advice before, during and after pregnancy as part of your maternity team.
- Advice about diabetes if you have carers that visit you at home.
- The opportunity to involve relatives, partners and friends in giving you support.
- The educational sessions and appointments you need.
- Information about managing your diabetes medication when you are ill.

IF YOU TAKE INSULIN YOU WILL LEARN[5]:

- How to inject yourself and how to store your insulin.
- How to dispose of syringes and needles.
- How to test your BG and your urine for ketones and what the results mean.
- How to recognise and treat low BG.

4 Diabetes UK (2000), *What Diabetes Care to Expect* (London: Diabetes UK).
5 Ibid.

You will also be given insulin supplies – or a prescription for insulin – and the equipment you need to give yourself insulin and test your BG.

IF YOUR DIABETES IS TREATED WITH TABLETS YOU WILL LEARN[6]:

- How to test your blood and urine for glucose and what the results mean.
- When low BG may happen and how to deal with it.

You will also be given a supply of your glucose-reducing tablets – or a prescription for them – and blood and urine testing equipment.

IF YOUR DIABETES IS MANAGED BY DIET YOU WILL[7]:

- Receive blood and urine glucose-testing equipment and be told how to interpret your results.

FACT: Your hospital diabetes clinic will provide your first prescription, then you'll need to order further prescriptions from your GP surgery. Prescriptions of insulin, needles, BG-lowering medication, lancets and test strips are free with an exemption certificate from your local health authority. You may have to buy a BG-testing meter.

---

6   Diabetes UK (2000), *What Diabetes Care to Expect*. (London: Diabetes UK).
7   Ibid.

What to expect when you see the diabetes nurse

Annual monitoring if you have Type 1 diabetes will involve having BG, blood pressure and weight measured and recording these with the result of your last HbA1c test to see if there are any changes. A urine sample will be taken to test for glucose, ketones and protein.

If you have Type 2 diabetes, the diabetes nurse will measure blood pressure and urine[8] to check for any kidney changes, especially if you have poor BG control. The nurse will also carry out a cardiovascular function check – heart and circulatory system – and diabetes complications risk assessment, as well as giving you measures to manage blood fats. You will start taking tablets (statins) to reduce cholesterol levels if necessary. You may also be advised to take a 75mg daily dose of aspirin to prevent blood clots.

What to expect when you see your diabetes consultant

You will periodically have an appointment for a consultation with your diabetes specialist – unless you have Type 2 diabetes and receive your care from your GP practice. Even if this is the case, there are certain things that you should expect from your appointment[9]:

- To receive regular health checks such as HbA1c blood testing for glucose levels, urine testing and foot examination.
- To be informed of changes in your condition that may lead to diabetic complications; to be advised of any changes in your care; to have test results simply explained in a way you can understand.
- To discuss lifestyle issues that may be affecting your BG control; to provide you with ongoing education about your diabetes; and to answer any questions you might have.

8   Diabetes UK (2000), *What Diabetes Care to Expect.* (London: Diabetes UK).
9   Ibid.

Arrive at your appointments prepared with a list of written questions so you can remind yourself if you get side-tracked; read as much as you can about diabetes, so you are confident, informed and in a position to discuss your condition. In addition, find out how much time you'll have with your consultant or other health professionals. Bring a sample of urine and your BG monitoring diary with you.

YOUR RESPONSIBILITIES AS A DIABETES TEAM MEMBER

Even though your diabetes care team is there to inform, guide and support you, diabetes is a health condition where 95 per cent of the management is down to you. As you are the person that is in charge of your diabetes, you must[10]:

- Be responsible for as much of your own day-to-day diabetes care as possible. This means finding out all you can about your condition to make the management easier.
- Make appropriate food choices and undertake regular exercise and BG monitoring.
- Check your feet daily, or as often as you can. (If you can't do it, ask someone else.)
- Ask for help to manage your diabetes if and when you need it, such as when you are ill with an infection or stomach upset.
- Know who, when and where to contact the people who can help you.
- Take on the diabetes-management advice you receive and ask your diabetes team for the information and advice you need. **Make a list** of things to ask so you don't forget.
- Go to your diabetes clinic appointments, and any others that will help you such as eye and foot care appointments.

10 Diabetes UK (2000), *What Diabetes Care to Expect.* (London: Diabetes UK.)

WHAT ABOUT IF I HAVE TO GO INTO HOSPITAL AND CAN'T BE IN CONTROL?

Going into hospital is always a worrying time, whether it's related to your diabetes or not. Once you are in hospital, your care is shared between you and the health professionals on the ward. It can be difficult to maintain good BG control when you're not living your normal lifestyle – your BG may be much higher because you're not physically active for a period of time. You will need to increase your insulin or BG-lowering medication to cover this inactivity, so your BG is as near-normal as possible – this will help you to heal more quickly, especially if you have had an operation. You should have the opportunity to discuss any concerns with a doctor or nurse before you are admitted to hospital, or once you are there. During your stay in hospital[11]:

- You will receive an explanation of your medical treatment while you are in hospital.
- You will be able to inform ward staff about your dietary needs, tablets or insulin treatment.
- You will be able to inform your hospital diabetes team of your admission.
- You will be able to do your own blood and urine glucose monitoring – and insulin injections – if you are well enough.
- Your insulin, if you take it, may be given in an intravenous drip with glucose if you are not allowed to eat before an operation. Your BG control will be managed by an anaesthetist during your operation.
- Your dosage of BG-lowering medication will change and you may be put on insulin temporarily.
- You should bring supplies of sweet foods to reverse low BG if you use insulin or sulphonylureas to treat your diabetes. Tell the nursing staff if you do have a hypo.
- Your diabetes control will be worse because you are not moving about, you are in a different environment and you may experience pain that can increase BG.

11 Diabetes UK (2000), *What Diabetes Care to Expect* (London: Diabetes UK).

FACT: The staff on hospital wards are very used to helping people with diabetes so don't worry – they will be familiar with what you have to do to manage your condition.

Case study: Mark

Mark King was admitted to hospital to have a hip replacement. He was worried about having to hand over control of his Type 1 diabetes to health professionals who didn't know him or his routine. When he was admitted, a nurse, Kay, came to find out about when Mark usually did his insulin injections and BG monitoring. Kay also explained Mark's surgical procedure and how his diabetes would be managed until he left hospital. Kay informed the hospital diabetes team of Mark's admission, told him when mealtimes were so he could give his insulin accordingly, and assured him that he would be seen only by staff fully trained in the care of patients with diabetes. Mark was advised about returning to his usual insulin treatment when he left hospital and that he would have regular check-ups. This personal care helped Mark to feel confident about managing his diabetes during his stay in hospital.

Case study: Shian

Shian Serei had Type 2 diabetes and a bad chest infection. Her GP arranged to admit her to hospital because she had ketones in her urine and high BG levels because of the infection. Shian was worried about going into hospital because she didn't speak English very well, but her sister spoke to Shian's diabetes nurse over the phone and she advised that Shian's sister attended when Shian was admitted so she could interpret and make sure Shian received culturally appropriate diabetes care while she was in hospital. This gave Shian peace of mind. Having her family members involved in her hospital diabetes care also helped Shian recover more quickly and she was able to go home a week later once her infection and diabetes were stabilised.

FACT: **If you have been waiting a long time for your hospital diabetes check-up or follow-up appointment, you should contact your GP so they can chase this up for you.**

How to make a complaint about your diabetes care[12]

If you have a complaint about the NHS diabetes care you receive in the UK, you should speak to your GP and/or your diabetes team who have a complaints procedure. You will be asked to put your complaint in writing and you will be told to contact *PALS* – the Patient and Liaison Service – who can act as a go-between as your complaint is investigated. This may take some time, but you will receive an outcome.

If the way your complaint is handled, or the reply you receive is not satisfactory to you, you can take the matter to your local Health Authority complaints office so that an impartial review panel can consider it. If this fails to resolve the issue, you can take the matter even further to the Health Service Ombudsman. Your local Community Health Council – CHC – can give you the details of how to contact the Health Service Ombudsman.

12 Diabetes UK (2000), *What Diabetes Care to Expect* (London: Diabetes UK).

Chapter 12

Young and Old

'The public needs to be shown that anyone can be affected by diabetes.'

Babies and small children with diabetes

Babies and toddlers with Type 1 diabetes

There are all sorts of practical challenges – on top of the health ones – if you have a baby or toddler with undiagnosed Type 1 diabetes. For example, developing language skills probably won't give your pre-schooler the vocabulary to tell you if he or she is feeling unwell. If your baby has not progressed to potty training, you won't be able to tell how much urine is being passed into their nappy; and if your baby has diarrhoea and vomiting and/or loses weight, you might think they have a tummy upset. Because of these factors, it may be some time before you receive a diagnosis of diabetes, by which time your baby could be very ill.

Once you have a diagnosis, your baby will be admitted to the *paediatric* intensive care unit at the hospital to begin insulin treatment, but it's important that you **don't blame yourself** – there is no way you could have known that your baby or toddler had undiagnosed diabetes.

FACT: Cases of Type 1 diabetes[1] are increasing, especially in children under 5 years old, with a recent 6.3-per-cent annual increase in cases compared to an overall increase of 3.4 per cent across all age groups.

---

1   Snouffer, E. B. (2017), 'Upsurge: The rise in Type 1 diabetes', *Diabetes Voice* 64(4), pp.22–5.

When you finally have a diagnosis, you will learn how to give your baby or pre-school child daily insulin and test their BG. It's fairly common for babies and toddlers to be resistant to their daily checks, and some will even find them distressing to go through – which can make doing them really hard for you. However, remember that your child **needs** to have insulin and BG checks – you aren't harming or hurting them, but helping them to stay healthy. Offer lots of reassuring cuddles afterwards, which will help both of you to feel better. You will also learn how to feed your baby regularly with the right food to prevent low BG.

Although the emphasis is on good control of BG in diabetes, this is less important for babies with the condition because the nervous system has not fully developed and therefore high BG levels can't affect it. Damage from high BG levels doesn't start to happen until just before the child reaches puberty. Aim to prevent frequent hypoglycaemia, which is what causes damage to the nerves rather than high BG. It's important to remember that small changes in the chemical balance of a baby's system cause illness very quickly. Aim to keep your baby's BG between 8.3 and 11.0 mmol/L.

FACT: Young people may experience a *honeymoon period* after Type 1 diabetes is diagnosed, where they need very little insulin to keep BG under control. Unfortunately, this doesn't last.

The honeymoon period will last longer in older children if the symptoms of Type 1 diabetes before diagnosis were mild rather than dramatic, and if the body's attack on the insulin-producing cells of the pancreas does not wipe out all insulin-producing cells as soon as they are formed. When the honeymoon period ends, BG levels rise again because insulin is no longer being produced. The diabetes team looking after your child will work out how much insulin is needed to control your child's condition. You will then be taught to:

- Recognise the signs of high and low BG and diabetic ketoacidosis – sickness and vomiting, rapid breathing, sleepiness/drowsiness, weakness.
- Give insulin – short-acting fits better with children's eating habits, which may include irregular mealtimes and not finishing everything they have been given.
- Test BG and urine ketone levels.
- Treat low BG with glucose or a glucagen injection kit.
- Feed a baby or child who has diabetes.
- React when your child is unwell with an illness other than diabetes.

Because your child can't carry out his or her own diabetes self-care, managing your baby or toddler's diabetes is very demanding, and can become even more stressful when you have to hand over that care to someone else for a while (if you're working, say). Toddlers learn to become more independent as they approach the time they go to school, but it's important to remember that calls for independence are not the same as capability! A young child still needs you to be in control of their management, with their own independence increasing slowly according to age, understanding and maturity.

FACT: Studies show that siblings of diabetic children can become jealous or demanding as a result of the extra attention the child with diabetes receives. Work together to include everyone in your child's diabetes care (meal planning together is a great way for everyone to be involved, for example) and praise all the work the siblings do to show that they are helping, too.

Type 2 diabetes in children

Although Type 2 diabetes is traditionally a condition seen in middle age, children as young as seven years of age are now also developing this disease[2]. Some children are more at risk than others. The reasons for insulin resistance developing in the very young are:

- Increased weight above normal childhood weight gain.
- A family history of insulin resistance and Type 2 diabetes.
- Being from a racial minority group, such as Southeast Asians, Native Americans, Pacific Islanders or African Americans.

The reason for identifying babies and children with insulin resistance as early as possible is to be able to advise that the family make lifestyle changes before the young person develops Type 2 diabetes. It's possible to reverse insulin resistance in the young with permanent diet, exercise and lifestyle changes, and to avoid Type 2 altogether – just as it is with adults.

FACT: **Children with any of the Type 2 risk factors should see a GP or practice nurse regularly to have their fasting BG measured.**

Care of children with diabetes at school

A school-age child can let you know how they feel, which makes hypos easier to detect. However, now that your child is not in your care during the day, BG control can become more difficult. The Department of Health says that children and young people spend a third of their daily lives at school and currently one in 550 school children has Type 1 diabetes; and 85 per cent of these have an HbA1c of above 7.7 per cent. This means that these children have diabetes that is not well controlled. School and nursery staff **must**

---

2   Temneanu, O. R., et al. (2016), 'Type 2 diabetes mellitus in children and adolescents: a relatively new clinical problem within pediatric medicine', *Journal of Medicine and Life* 9(3), pp. 235–9.

understand the importance of managing diabetes in the children in their care.

FACT: **Diabetes health professionals can educate and train school staff so they can support your child while he or she is away from home.**

Children with Type 1 need to have multiple daily injections of insulin throughout the day to keep BG levels as normal as possible. One of these injections will be at lunchtime and most children between 9 and 16 years old will do this themselves. If not, though, either a parent or a member of school staff has to give the injection. Bear in mind that needle use has to be supervised closely in school for health and safety reasons (the same goes for BG testing with lancets). If you aren't able to come into school to administer the injection, it's very important that at least one member of school staff knows exactly what to do and when. Children of 11 years old or older who have had Type 1 for a while can usually inject their own insulin, but they will still need a member of staff present.

An insulin pump is attached to the body 24/7 and if your child uses this way of delivering their insulin, they will go to see the school nurse at lunchtime to have their BG monitored and to get their insulin bolus – dose – before they eat. Insulin pumps have a lock function to stop the pump giving a bolus of insulin unless it's specifically needed. This prevents children from pressing buttons on the pump and giving unnecessary insulin that could cause low BG.

Pumps can also work with a glucose sensor to warn of high and low glucose levels if your child has Type 1 diabetes that is very difficult to control – known as *brittle diabetes*. This means that all of your child's teachers need to be aware that the pump alarm may sound during lessons and that your child will need to go to the school nurse to receive glucose, or a bolus of insulin if BG is very high. But if it's a hypo, the child should be treated for low BG **where**

they are, not sent anywhere else – especially if the reading shows a very low BG.

FACT: School staff are bound by a common duty-of-care law to make sure children with diabetes are healthy and safe. This law covers administering medication as well as action in an emergency, including the treatment of hypoglycaemia.

The ideal situation for a child with diabetes is for BG results at school to be as good as when they're at home. Schools and Local Education Authorities – LEAs – are obliged **not** to treat children with diabetes less favourably than those without diabetes unless they can provide a valid reason. This means that schools can't state that they will refuse to administer medication of any kind or insist that parents must come into school to do this for their child. It can be very difficult and worrying for a parent to hand over the care of their child to the school during the day – the school **must** be fully aware of their role in your child's daily diabetes management.

Case study: Ben

Susan Parker's son Ben was diagnosed with Type 1 diabetes when he was 6 years old. Susan worked full time but came into the school to give Ben his insulin every lunchtime for three months. She then made it clear to the school that it was their responsibility to manage Ben's diabetes during the day while he was in their care. Susan spoke with Ben's Children's Diabetes Nurse Specialist – CDNS – and they both visited Ben's school to discuss the staff's responsibilities in administering Ben's necessary injections. Once the school was clear on their role in Ben's diabetes care, Susan found there were no more problems.

Below is a list of knowledge and skills that your child's school should have to support a child with diabetes of up to 11 years of age[3]:

- Awareness to test BG if a child says they feel unwell, as symptoms of low BG can be confused with high BG. It's important to test BG **before** any glucose or insulin is given.

- Ability to recognise the symptoms of low BG as young children may not be able to do this, especially if they are playing or concentrating in class.

- Ability to treat low BG of less than 4.0 mmol/L as young children may not be able to do this themselves, especially if they are disorientated. The child **should not** be sent anywhere else to treat their hypo.

- Ability to act quickly on the child's behalf, as young children may not feel confident and able to approach an adult in authority.

- Ability to supervise and support BG testing as young children need to be reminded to wash their hands and may need help with the testing process, especially when interpreting the results.

- Ability to supervise the child giving insulin via a pen or pump.

- Ability to help the child calculate the carbohydrate content of meals and awareness that a child may eat more if they share food with others, or less if they drop food or don't want to eat part of their meal.

- Ability to plan ahead for exercise so that glucose is taken or is available, as children may forget or be distracted.

- If the child uses pump therapy, the ability to help the child with numeracy skills. When calculating insulin or programming an insulin pump, the position of the decimal point on insulin delivery is crucial – such as the difference between 10.0 units and 1.0 unit of insulin.

- Knowledge of how to **suspend** insulin delivery on the pump when the child has a low BG – although there is an auto-suspend function

---

3   Diabetes UK (2018), 'Diabetes in schools: Information for teachers and staff'. See www.diabetes,org,uk/guide-to-diabetes/your-child-diabetes/schools/schools-staff.

on some models – as their own ability may be impaired, and when/how to **resume** insulin delivery once BG has returned to normal.

* Ability to recognise equipment problems, such as a no delivery of insulin alarm; understanding the meanings of pump alarms, and knowing who to contact.

FACT: Schools do not currently test children's urine for ketones in cases of illness and when there is very high BG, so parents have to come into school to do this.

FACT: Schools do not currently support the use of glucagen injection kits in cases of severe hypoglycaemia and will phone the emergency services to do this.

Case study: Lisa

Peter Davis received a phone call at work to say that his 10-year-old daughter, Lisa, was having a bad hypo. She'd been running around the playground with her friends and collapsed during an afternoon class, shaking and sweating. Lisa's teacher called an ambulance because she'd been told this was an emergency situation. Peter Davis quickly left work, stopped off at home to grab a glucagen injection kit, and rushed to Lisa's school. When Peter arrived, he found Lisa had been taken to the school nurse's room because the other children were frightened by her behaviour. When the paramedic arrived, he said he wasn't trained to give glucagen. Peter was very angry and pushed past them to give Lisa the injection he had brought from home before she dropped into unconsciousness. Peter did a BG test and found that Lisa was 2.5 mmol/L. After ten minutes, she became more coherent and her next BG was 5.0 mmol/L. Peter took Lisa home, although she was fine after her severely low BG had been treated. Peter warns other parents to always take a glucagen injection kit along to the school if the school phones to say a child with diabetes is ill.

Hypo-busting tips

When you tighten your child's BG control there's less glucose in the blood, so hypos can happen more often. This is frequently the case at bedtime, after your child has digested an evening meal, but there is still insulin working in the bloodstream. When your child goes to bed, make sure that you[4]:

- Give them a bedtime snack, such as a couple of plain biscuits.
- Check your child's BG before they go to sleep.
- Ask your child if they have experienced symptoms of low BG during the night, such as nightmares or headaches. Do an occasional BG test at 3 a.m.
- Know if your child hasn't eaten all of their meal.
- Give your child extra carbohydrate to eat before exercising.
- Tell your child's school who to contact in an emergency.

FACT: Frequent hypoglycaemia in children does not damage a child's brain.

4   Jarvis, S. & Rubin, A. (2003), *Diabetes for Dummies* (Chichester: John Wiley & Sons Ltd.), p.223.

It is helpful to take your child to the supermarket so they can learn about food labels and foods that are high in calories, fats and carbohydrates, especially if you have been told by their diabetes consultant that they need to lose some weight. When I was first diagnosed at age ten, although I was thin because I wasn't 'allowed' to eat certain foods, this made them very desirable to me. I would take a detour to the shops on my way to school and spend my pocket money on crisps and chocolate. As a child, I thought I was getting back at the doctors, not realising that I was on a restricted diet for a reason.

Having diabetes now is completely different because of Dose Adjustment For Normal Eating – DAFNE – so children don't have to miss out on the occasional treat, especially if they have low BG or are about to exercise. This makes it easier if you also have other non-diabetic children who don't have to watch their diet. Make sure that you never use food – such as a trip to a fast-food restaurant, or other high-calorie, unhealthy foods – as a reward so that your child knows it's better to eat a banana for carbohydrate than crisps.

Diet and exercise[5]

- Nutritional needs for children change constantly. As your child grows, they will be eating much more food for cell growth, so it's important to keep in touch with the dietician in your child's diabetes team.
- Children can be very physically active, especially when playing with friends. Make sure they are aware that running around can cause hypos.
- Help your child make the right food choices and let them decide that what they want to eat then fits with those choices. They are more likely to eat meals if they've chosen them themselves.
- Children should have a certain amount of fat in their diet as they grow so children under 2 years old – or those who won't eat properly – should be given full-fat milk, yoghurt and cheese rather than low-fat varieties.

5   Jarvis, S. & Rubin, A. (2003), *Diabetes for Dummies* (Chichester: John Wiley & Sons Ltd.), pp.228–30.

- High-fibre foods are not suitable for young children. Give them refined carbohydrates, such as white rice, pasta or bread; unsweetened cereals; potatoes and fruit instead.
- Make sure your child knows how to make healthy food choices at school – for example, jacket potato instead of chips – and why this is important for their health.
- It's normal to worry about what your child eats and how much physical activity they do when they're at school or visiting a friend's house. The hospital dietician can help by giving suggestions.

FACT: Buying 'diabetic' chocolate, sweets, cakes or ice cream is a waste of time. They are usually more expensive, don't always taste nice, and still contain sugar or a sweetener that can cause diarrhoea. It's better for your child to eat normal foods in measured amounts and take the insulin dosage necessary for the carbohydrate content.

TEENAGERS WITH TYPE 1 DIABETES

Most cases of Type 1 diabetes happen during the teenage years. If it was diagnosed earlier than this, your child will have avoided the risk of complications, but once they reach 13 years of age, BG must be controlled. Diabetes self-management is difficult at any age, but being a teenager makes this even more challenging. Teenagers may not consider long-term complications, and can be unwilling or forgetful or preoccupied when it comes to testing their BG regularly. There are lots of issues for this age group that make managing diabetes difficult, such as:

- Hormonal changes increasing BG because of insulin resistance.
- Increased risk of ketosis in association with high BG.
- A desire to be independent.

- Trying to remain and identify within the group-thinking/actions of their close friends – peer pressure.
- Resisting authority.
- Changing from a child – paediatric – to adult diabetes clinic for their care.

Your child's desire to become independent is probably one of the biggest challenges you will face as a parent. Although this might seem like a good idea – especially letting them take control of their own diabetes – you should hold on to the reins of diabetes control until you judge your child is mature enough to self-manage their condition:

- Setting clear rules that you oversee inevitably means better BG control for your child.
- Your child may want to act like friends who don't have diabetes, meaning he or she misses injections or BG tests.
- Teenagers may be unable/unwilling to interpret BG results and act upon them.
- Weight issues, especially in girls, may start to trouble your child. There is a condition called *diabulimia* – thought to affect one-third of women and young girls, and some boys with Type 1 diabetes – where insulin is reduced or completely omitted to induce ketoacidosis and rapid weight loss. This is done very secretively and parents may not even know it's happening repeatedly, putting the young person at risk of diabetic ketoacidosis and chronic, severe complications such as eye, nerve and kidney disease.

FACT: The medical profession does not recognise diabulimia as an eating disorder, despite the fact that it's deliberate diabetes mis-management.

Case study: Alissa

Alissa Thomas developed Type 1 diabetes when she was 11 years old and soon found out that, when she was ill with diabetic ketoacidosis, she could lose about 6.4kg in a week. Alissa was admitted to hospital several times with DKA because she had repeated chest infections, and discovered that DKA is owing to hyperglycaemia and a lack of insulin. As Alissa grew older, she became more and more aware of her weight and body image. Although she was underweight for her height, she began cutting down on the amount of insulin she took so that she felt sick and had little appetite. Alissa's parents knew she'd lost weight each time she was ill, but they began to notice that she skipped meals and was losing weight when she was apparently well. They took her to her doctor and tests showed that Alissa had ketones in her urine. The doctor explained that Alissa already had early signs of eye disease associated with continually high BG levels and that if she carried on under-dosing on her insulin, she could damage other vital organs as well. Alissa realised how much damage she was doing and began looking after her diabetes properly, although she admits that it's still very tempting to try and lose weight this way from time to time.

FACT: Diabetic ketoacidosis is a serious *acute* medical condition and it is fatal in 10 per cent of cases – especially if there is another illness to complicate DKA. Don't be tempted to reduce or omit your insulin to try and lose weight quickly.

Case study: Drew

Drew Morris was 14 years old when he started being bullied about both his diabetes and his weight. Although people with Type 1 diabetes tend to be lean, Drew was slightly overweight for his height. When he was being teased, he tried to shrug it off, but the comments really got to him and he began trying to take control of the situation by under-dosing on the amount of insulin he was taking. This was Drew's way of taking action, although he didn't realise how dangerous it was. He noticed that his BG tests were much higher because he had less insulin in his bloodstream and he also found that he was losing weight steadily. Drew's parents thought this was because he was attending an after-school sports club, but this wasn't the case. Eventually, Drew became very ill with DKA and was admitted to hospital. He underwent tests and it was discovered that he had early kidney damage related to his high BG levels over time. Drew felt guilty, especially as his mother was telling him it was such a shame that diabetes had affected him like this; Drew knew he could have prevented this damage. From that day, he decided to manage his diabetes properly to prevent any further deterioration in kidney function.

It can be difficult to get young people to participate in looking after their diabetes. Hospital diabetes teams – paediatric diabetes clinics – caring for teenagers with the condition now use technology to try and engage teenagers in their diabetes care[6]. Hospitals use methods such as texting reminders to test BG to a child's mobile, and asking young patients to text their blood results back to be recorded (as well as estimated monthly HbA1c values), which have proved successful. Using modern technology in this way has been successful

6   Franklin, V. (2016), 'Influences on technology use and efficacy in Type 1 diabetes', *Journal of Diabetes Science and Technology*. org/10.1177/1932296816639315.

because it breaks down barriers between the hospital diabetes clinic and the teenager, helping teenagers to feel that their diabetes management is relevant to their everyday life.

Case study: Joel

Joel Pinder-King was 15 years old with Type 1 diabetes from age six. He tended not to take it too seriously, doing the same things his friends did without making sure he had glucose with him. Joel also sometimes forgot to do his insulin injections, or took them at the wrong times. Joel's BG results were usually either too low or too high because of the way he managed his condition. His diabetes nurse suggested he texted his BG results to a particular web address that would store the information and allow experts to analyse the results. Joel also agreed that he was happy to receive text alerts to remind him to take his insulin throughout the day. After three months with the new system, Joel's diabetes control was much better. He also received clinic appointment reminders; had his diabetes-related questions answered quickly (including discovering that he shouldn't inject his insulin through his clothes); and discovered that other people felt the same way about their diabetes.

STUDENTS MANAGING DIABETES AWAY FROM HOME

There comes a time when your child will need to be independent and you will need to pass their diabetes control fully over to them. By this time your child will have been doing their own injections and BG testing for a number of years, managing their condition alongside you and knowing what they need to do and when. Leaving home, though, is the first time he or she will become fully independent – without the reassurance of you being on hand to step in and react if something goes wrong.

Very little has been written about the experiences of young adults with diabetes who leave home to go to college or university – so instead talk through the implications together and try to establish an action plan that your child is confident about following on his or her own. Make sure he or she realises that there will be a big challenge ahead: juggling diabetes self-management, along with establishing his or her own identity, and dealing with peer group and authority pressures, as well as hormonal variations that can stop insulin working as well. To exacerbate the upheaval, your child may need to transfer from paediatric to adult diabetes care at this time.

FACT: A 70-per-cent rise in Type 1 diabetes is predicted in young people aged 15 and above over the next few years.

Balancing diabetes and further education

Students often feel that they don't receive adequate support from their college/university and their diabetes team to be able to manage the demands of further education and diabetes self-management. All students experience stress, but this can complicate diabetes by increasing BG levels. Being in a different environment with a change in routine can also make injecting insulin several times a day, BG testing and eating on time much more difficult, but after a while the new routine will become easier and your child will get to know when BG is more likely to become low so they can eat some glucose tablets if they can't get any food at the time. Lecture times may not be the only issue: your young adult may not want to attract the attention of others by insisting they have to eat or inject.

Case study: Emma

Emma Khan was 18 years old with Type 1 diabetes. She was in her first year at university and had found the change very difficult because university was not as flexible as her school used to be in letting her go out of class to test her BG or inject her insulin. Some days, the lectures were all day from 9 a.m. until 6 p.m., with an hour for lunch at midday, and on others they were 9 a.m. until 1 p.m. with the afternoon off. Emma didn't have time to test her BG between lectures and she found it embarrassing to make an issue of this. She eventually got into a routine of not testing her BG when she was with other people and having less insulin to avoid hypogly-caemia, although she knew it was dangerous. Emma tested her BG only when she felt sick, affecting her ability to work or concentrate.

Case study: Paige

Paige Wells was in her second year at university and found that managing her Type 1 diabetes was not at all easy when she was away from home. Paige felt that despite the fact she had told the university about her diabetes, and her diabetes team that she was at university, she inevitably had to manage on her own. She informed one of her tutors that she needed a break during a three-hour exam to check her BG and he replied that Paige should have made sure she could sit through the exam without interruption. On another occasion, Paige tried to organise an appointment with her new, adult diabetes team, but they said she needed a referral from her GP who was miles away in her home town. Her paediatric team also said they could no longer see her as she must transfer to the adult clinic. Paige felt stuck in the middle, abandoned with no one to help or support her. She added that this must be a common prob-lem for young people with diabetes.

Hypoglycaemia is a massive worry when you have diabetes and you are away from home, especially if you don't feel confident you can deal with it. I recall a particularly horrible incident when I was visiting a university where no one knew me – attending a three-day diabetes conference, surrounded by diabetes consultants from all over the world! Having crossed a rather busy road, I developed a very severe and unexpected hypo with no warning signs and collapsed unconscious in some bushes. After a while, I regained consciousness and managed to stagger to the porter's lodge where I dropped into unconsciousness again. I was extremely lucky that the porter phoned one of the course tutors – an expert in hypoglycaemia – who came rushing over with a glucagen injection to bring me round. This example is what people who take insulin fear most – losing control and having to rely on someone else to know what to do.

Adverse diabetes management strategies

This fear of the disabling effects of hypoglycaemia causes some people to deliberately take less insulin so that their BG is too high rather than too low. This tactic is especially true of students who want to fit in and don't want the fuss and embarrassment of having a public hypo.

Case study: Vin

Vin Gupta says that she hates having hypos because they take away her feeling of control. She explained that it's impossible to tell everyone you have to deal with what a hypo is and how to treat it. Vin's doctor told her she had to take responsibility for her own diabetes, especially because she was away from home at university. Because she was continually worried, Vin found it easier to have higher BG levels so she didn't have a hypo, although she knew this tactic increased the chance of developing long-term complications from having poor BG control. Vin hated being ill and people fussing over her, especially when they didn't understand what was wrong and she couldn't make herself understood when she had low glucose levels. Vin also felt that people didn't understand why her personality altered when she was hypo, so this was something she tried to avoid; she kept her BG around 12 mmol/L, saying she felt better mentally than when her glucose level was 5.0–6.0 mmol/L.

Reduced participation in social events

Another issue for students away from home at college or university is the feeling that their diabetes has affected their ability to enjoy social events. This ties in with wanting to appear normal and avoid hypos in a social situation. Feeling able to join in has many issues attached to it, such as: having to restrict or avoid alcohol when there is pressure to drink; having to watch BG levels if dancing is involved; not knowing the carbohydrate values of foods on offer at parties; and having to act and draw attention if hypos do happen, especially if friends feel they have to be responsible in this situation. Eating out and injecting before the meal can also be difficult, so some feel that it's easier to just enjoy themselves and not worry about diabetes. This strategy won't do any harm if it's only once in a while, but if it happens several times a week, this is not good diabetes self-management.

In summary

- Many students – if they are being honest – feel that they don't have good control of their diabetes at college or university.
- Students with diabetes often have problems balancing their healthcare and their educational needs.
- Rather than have a hypo in a classroom or social situation, some students with diabetes would rather have a higher BG to avoid this risk.
- Many students with diabetes feel they receive little support from either their college/university or diabetes team, and they may have problems even getting an appointment during the holidays or when they are away from home studying.

- Individuals with diabetes may not wish to tell their peers about their condition because it's a hidden disability and they don't want to appear different.
- Students with diabetes may not join in with social events for fear of embarrassment over hypos, or they may 'ignore' their diabetes so they can have a good time with friends.

It is difficult to overcome these problems, especially if your young adult doesn't talk to you or the college/university about them. Paediatric diabetes teams could liaise with adult clinics to make the changeover easier for young adults, and this may help to identify difficulties such as arranging appointments when your young adult is at home. In this way, they will be able to discuss any problems they have had during their time away from home.

ISSUES FOR OLDER PEOPLE WITH DIABETES

According to the World Health Organisation, by 2025 the number of people in the UK in their eighties and nineties will have doubled. Older people with diabetes have a 70-per-cent higher rate of hospital admission. It's important to remember that older people might have had Type 1 diabetes all their life; they may have developed Type 2 diabetes in their forties or fifties; or they may even be newly diagnosed. Because rates of Type 2 are escalating, a distinction between Type 1 and Type 2 is no longer made and 'diabetes' has become a general term for everyone with the condition. Health professionals can also assume that your diabetes is Type 2 because you are attending a diabetes clinic full of people with Type 2, rather than understanding that you've had Type 1 since childhood.

FACT: The Department of Health has stated that older people should be treated as individuals and are enabled to make choices about their diabetes care.

If an older person has not lived their life with Type 1 diabetes, or developed Type 2 in their middle years, they may develop 'elderly onset' Type 2. Here, insulin is produced at a normal rate, but it doesn't work as well, increasing BG levels. Type 2 diabetes is very common in older people because insulin is less effective, even when there is no obesity and the person is active. Because of this, BG levels become much higher than normal after meals.

Older people may not complain of the symptoms of Type 2 diabetes, or symptoms may go unnoticed as they happen over many years. Particular symptoms of Type 2 in older people may be[7]:

- Loss of appetite.
- Weakness.
- Weight loss.
- Loss of bladder control – usually owing to the prostate gland pressing on the bladder in men and bladder and kidney infections in women.

FACT: Older people with untreated Type 2 diabetes may not have thirst as a symptom as their ability to feel thirst is altered.

While many older people with diabetes manage their condition very well, certain problems connected with older age can affect their control of BG:

Mental functioning

Mental function in older persons may be impaired, making it difficult to access the mental agility required for following a specific diet and medication regime, and testing BG regularly, if necessary. (Regular BG testing may not be the case if diabetes is diagnosed in an elderly person, as the emphasis is not

---

7 Jarvis, S. & Rubin, A. (2003), *Diabetes for Dummies* (Chichester: John Wiley & Sons Ltd.), p.234.

on keeping BG under control because complications are unlikely to develop within that person's lifetime.)

Studies have shown that there is a link between the development of dementia and having either Type 1 or Type 2 diabetes[8], making it much harder to carry out diabetes self-care tasks. If dementia or Alzheimer's disease is diagnosed, tests to determine mental functioning can show whether the person is able to live alone, or whether they need a carer to visit, sheltered housing or nursing-home care.

Diet

Many older people with diabetes are able to care for themselves and may have problems only associated with getting proper nutrition. Preparing healthy meals can also be difficult because the older person has:

- A lower income.
- Poor vision.
- Poor appetite owing to decreased taste and smell.
- Arthritis or tremors, making food preparation difficult.
- Poor teeth or a dry mouth.
- Depression so that they don't feel like eating.
- A sense that they are too old to worry about caring for diabetes.

One or many of these problems may mean that the elderly person has an inadequate diet and poor diabetes control. In the UK, Social Services can make sure one nutritious, cooked meal suited to the diabetes diet is delivered to the individual's home every day. Some areas also provide meal choices for different ethnic backgrounds, and private companies provide meals by daily or weekly deliveries.

Exercise

Exercise as a way to reduce BG may be limited in the elderly. Because older people are more likely to have coronary heart disease, arthritis, eye disease,

8   Jarvis, S. & Rubin, A. (2003), *Diabetes for Dummies* (Chichester: John Wiley & Sons Ltd.), p.234.

neuropathy and reduced blood flow in the feet and legs, any exercise must be gentle. The charity Help the Aged runs local groups that allow the individual to participate in gentle exercise, and also to socialise with other people.

FACT: One in four older people in care homes has diabetes.

Eyesight

Eye disease is more likely to occur in older people who have diabetes. Cataracts, *macular degeneration* and glaucoma, as well as diabetic retinopathy, are all more prevalent in elderly sufferers. Despite this, one third of older people have never had their eyes examined, meaning these eye conditions are not diagnosed and treated early on[9]. The vast majority of cases of diabetes-related blindness can be prevented with early treatment, so always go for an eye test, even if you think there's nothing wrong.

Urinary and sexual problems

Older people with diabetes are often affected by urinary and sexual health problems[10]. The bladder muscles can become paralysed so that urine can't be passed and, when the bladder becomes too full, the urine flows out. Mobility problems may also make it difficult to get to the toilet on time, and spasms in the bladder muscle may push urine out of the body. These problems can also cause frequent infections of the urinary tract.

9   Jarvis, S. & Rubin, A. (2003), *Diabetes for Dummies* (Chichester: John Wiley & Sons Ltd.), p.235.
10 Ibid., p.236.

More than 60 per cent of men over seventy who have diabetes also have erectile dysfunction and 50 per cent have no desire to have sex[11]. It's thought that older men are likely to have blocked blood vessels, affecting blood flow to the penis. Various medications taken by older men may also affect sexual function. Report any problems like this to your GP so that you can have the cause investigated and treated.

Medication

If you are elderly and can't use diet and exercise to control your BG, your diabetes care team will consider giving you glucose-lowering medication. While this solves one problem, it may present others, such as[12]:

- Taking the wrong dosage of tablets if poor eyesight is a problem.
- Confusion over what the tablets are for and why they are important if there is cognitive impairment.
- Difficulty with getting the child-proof bottle open to take the tablets when there is arthritis or infirmity.
- Problems with different medications reacting with one another.
- The presence of liver or kidney impairment meaning the medication effects last longer.
- Poor appetite meaning the individual has frequently low BG.

> FACT: A study of 113 older people with Type 2 diabetes showed that 90 per cent felt their BG-lowering medication was effective and necessary, but 60 per cent were also worried about the long-term effects of their tablets; 25 per cent felt some diabetes medications were over-prescribed by doctors.

11 Jarvis, S. & Rubin, A. (2003), *Diabetes for Dummies* (Chichester: John Wiley & Sons Ltd.), p.236.
12 Ibid., p.231.

When an older person who is prescribed BG-lowering tablets moves from looking after themselves to going into a care home, their dosages may need altering if they have not been taking the medication when they have been told to, or in the right amounts.

CARING FOR PEOPLE WITH DIABETES

Like all *chronic* health conditions, diabetes affects the relationship between couples and families. It's thought that the emotional costs of living with someone with diabetes are high, especially with Type 1 because of the mood swings associated with low BG, as well as feelings of irritation and frustration and the restrictions diabetes can impose on lifestyle – for everyone[13].

When a child or a young adult develops diabetes, it becomes a family condition, involving everyone in the need to follow a particular diet (as much as possible for inclusivity, without making anyone feel they're missing out, particularly siblings) and understand diabetes care, the implications of something going wrong, and what to do if it does.

Current thinking suggests that living with and caring for someone with diabetes can present significant mental and emotional challenges, including such things as being hyper-vigilant of the diabetic person's mood; sensing hypo just by tone of voice or behaviour; and encouraging and supporting self-care activities, among others. When the person with diabetes has to provide information about their condition to health professionals, this greatly increases their partner's understanding of how that person copes with their diabetes and this, in turn, helps the partner/carer cope better. This involvement by another person also helps the individual with diabetes to manage their condition and carry out their self-care tasks. This knowledge of a partner's health problems is known as '*condition specific*', meaning that they can take over diabetes management if necessary, such as during a hypo.

---

13 Johnson, N. L. & Melton, S. T. (2015), 'Partner perspectives on life with a person with Type 1 diabetes'. See theplaidjournal.com/index.php/com/article/view/48/32.

FACT: Knowledge and support from partners can improve diabetes self-management, but the nature of that support very much depends on the nature of the relationship.

Case study: John

Kathy Goldstein had been married to her husband, John, for twenty-two years. He had Type 1 diabetes when they met, so Kathy felt she had never known any different. John developed sight difficulties ten years later and relied on Kathy when they went shopping to read labels and to do the driving. Kathy felt that their relationship had changed from one where she relied on John to earn a wage and pay the bills to one in which she was a carer. She didn't mind this, but could see how some marriages might be affected by the progression of any chronic disease in one partner. Kathy felt it was important for John to know he had her support, and for her to suggest ways of dealing with certain life situations and diabetes-related problems that John hadn't thought of, like asking his diabetes nurse about getting a calibrated insulin syringe for the blind to overcome the difficulties he had in drawing up his insulin dosages.

Some partners feel that diabetes represents a third person in the relationship, and even a presence that cuts them out of their partner's life in some way. This is especially the case when the person with diabetes speaks to others with the condition, discussing shared experiences and being members of the 'diabetes club'. Although diabetes is something that you have to deal with yourself, support from others with and without the condition is really necessary to help you cope and manage as well as possible – make sure your partner knows that however much you need to talk to others who understand what it's like to have diabetes, you also need his or her support to help you manage your condition in your day-to-day lives.

Case study: Lynn

Keith Marshall didn't give his partner Lynn's diabetes another thought when they were younger because she could drive, work and look after herself and the house. When Lynn became pregnant in her late-twenties, Keith was concerned that her Type 1 diabetes would affect the baby, but because they were both still young, he didn't worry too much. Lynn had severe problems with her BG control during her pregnancy and she became more and more dependent on Keith to help around the house. Unfortunately, Lynn then had a miscarriage and she and Keith drifted apart when she really needed his support. Eventually, they split up because Keith blamed Lynn – and her diabetes – for losing the baby.

FACT: Partners like to feel they have some control over the condition too so that if the person can't do their insulin or a blood test, their partner can take on the role of carer and knows what to do.

Case study: Rav

Rav Nadim would get very irritated when his wife, Pria, invited her friends and family around to have a 'Type 2 diabetes party', where Pria would make carbohydrate-counted snacks and buy sugar-free drinks. Pria had four aunties with Type 2 and two friends that she'd met at diabetes clinic, and she enjoyed exchanging recipes and information with them. Although Pria carried on arranging these get-togethers every couple of months, she wished Rav would join in and support her in having to live with Type 2. Pria made special meals for herself while the rest of the family ate as much as they liked, which upset her. It was difficult to come to a compromise because Rav wanted Pria to eat what she'd cooked for the family, and Pria wanted Rav to understand her condition – that she had to watch what she ate as she controlled her diabetes through diet, exercise and medication. In the end, Pria's diabetes nurse was able to speak to Rav and explain the condition and the importance of diet to control BG. Rav was more supportive after this, explaining that he hadn't been *asked* to be involved in any of Pria's diabetes care or management.

It's important that everyone – health professionals, families and people with diabetes themselves – recognise that the person with diabetes is not the only one who has to deal with it. Because of this, both the person with diabetes *and* their partner might find it helpful to talk to other people who are going through the same problems. Involving a person's partner or other family members in diabetes discussions is reassuring for the individual with the condition, and also inclusive for the family themselves.

Recipes

'It's important that you enjoy your food!'

When a person is diagnosed with diabetes, and once they've been taught what they should and shouldn't be eating, it can be difficult to think of meal solutions that won't drastically increase BG levels. If you really want to get into diabetes-friendly cooking in a serious way there are many excellent cookbooks available that cover this subject – just make sure that the recipes in them by and large contain ingredients that you would want to cook.

Over the following pages, I have shared some of my favourite recipe suggestions for breakfast, lunch, dinner and treats. I've included the carbohydrate and calorie content of each meal, the sugar, fat and salt content, and how much of the daily five recommended portions of fruit or veg each contains. However, if you have food intolerances or allergies, make sure you stick only to what you know is safe for you to eat.

BREAKFAST SOLUTIONS

FRUITY PORRIDGE WITH TOASTED SEEDS

Serves 2

Preparation time: 15 minutes

Cooking time: 10 minutes

One serving contains 34.6g carbohydrate; 219 calories; 17.0g sugars;
5.8g fat; less than 0.1g salt; and half a portion of fruit.

Ingredients:

50g ready-to-eat dried apricots

150ml orange or apple juice

50g porridge oats

15g seeds such as pumpkin

Method:

1. Place the apricots in a small saucepan and cover with the fruit juice. Bring to the boil and simmer for 5 minutes.

2. Set the apricots aside for 10 minutes, then place them in a food processor/blender and blend to a purée.

3. Place the oats in a small saucepan and cover with 600ml of water. Place over a low heat to cook for 3–4 minutes. Meanwhile, toast the seeds under a medium grill.

4. Stir half the apricot purée into the porridge and divide between two bowls. Top with equal amounts of the toasted seeds and a swirl of purée.

POTATO PATTIES

Makes 12

Preparation time: 10 minutes

Cooking time: 25 minutes

Each patty contains 9.6g carbohydrate; 67 calories;

less than 0.5g sugars; 1.8g fat; and 0.2g salt.

Ingredients:

450g potatoes, peeled and chopped

3 eggs

Freshly grated nutmeg, to taste

50g self-raising flour

A little sunflower oil, for frying

Salt and freshly ground black pepper

Method:

1. Boil the potatoes for 10–12 minutes, or until soft. Drain and mash well, or press through a potato ricer. Leave to cool completely, then stir through beaten eggs (one whole egg and two yolks), nutmeg and flour and season well with salt and pepper.

2. Whisk two egg whites until they form soft peaks, then gently fold into the potato mixture. Heat a little oil in a non-stick frying pan, form the mixture into 12 patties and cook in batches until golden brown on both sides (approximately 2–3 minutes).

3. Set aside each batch on a piece of kitchen paper to absorb any excess oil and keep warm until you're ready to serve.

TASTY TOASTIES

Serves 4

Preparation time: 10 minutes

Cooking time: 10 minutes

Each toastie contains 35.3g carbohydrate; 294 calories; 3.3g sugars;

11g fat; 1.6g salt; and 1 portion of vegetables.

Ingredients:

1 wholemeal baguette, cut into 16 1.5cm-thick slices

8 cherry tomatoes, halved

1 red pepper, cored, seeded and thinly sliced

4 mushrooms, sliced

1 slice of lean ham, cut into strips

70g cooked spinach, water squeezed out

2 spring onions, finely sliced

2 eggs, scrambled

75g reduced-fat mature Cheddar cheese, finely grated

Method:

1. Heat your grill to medium and toast the baguette slices until golden on both sides. Allow to cool. (You could use the cooling time to prepare your toppings, if you haven't already.)

2. Use the remaining ingredients other than the cheese to top the slices of baguette – combine them according to your taste and preferences, making a few options.

3. Sprinkle each topped slice with a little grated Cheddar, then place them back under the grill until the cheese is golden and bubbling. Serve immediately.

MINI BERRY PANCAKES

Makes 10 pancakes

Preparation time: 10 minutes

Cooking time: 15–20 minutes

Each mini-pancake (74g) contains 16.3g carbohydrate; 100 calories;
2.8g sugars; 1.8g fat; 0.2g salt; and half a portion of fruit.

Ingredients:

200g wholemeal flour

1 tsp baking powder

1 medium egg, beaten

250ml skimmed milk

1 tsp vanilla extract

200g blueberries

2 tsp sunflower oil

1 tsp sugar substitute

Method:

1. Mix the flour and baking powder in a bowl.

2. In a separate bowl, beat together the egg, milk and vanilla extract.

3. Make a well in the middle of the flour, then gradually stir in the egg and milk mixture until you get a smooth batter.

4. Ideally, leave to stand for a few minutes before cooking.

5. Lightly crush half the blueberries with a fork and mix these into the batter along with the remaining whole blueberries.

6. Add a little oil to a non-stick frying-pan, then add spoonfuls of the batter to the pan making sure the blueberries are evenly distributed.

7. Cook the pancakes on a medium heat for 2–3 minutes then turn them and cook for a further 2 minutes. The pancakes are ready to turn when you see bubbles appearing on the surface. Sprinkle with a little sugar substitute before serving with a dash of lemon juice.

QUICK AND EASY APPLE AND CINNAMON PORRIDGE

Serves 1

Preparation time: 2 minutes

Cooking time: 2 minutes

Each serving contains 34g carbohydrate; 202 calories; 37g fat;

10.2g sugars; 0.01g salt; and 1 portion of fruit.

Ingredients:

35g porridge oats

1 tsp sugar substitute

1 tsp cinnamon, and a pinch for the top

1 small apple, cored and chopped finely

25ml semi-skimmed milk

Method:

1. Put the oats, sweetener, cinnamon and apple in a mug.

2. Add 100ml of water and cook on full power (800 watts) for 2 minutes.

3. Add the milk, mix and sprinkle with a little cinnamon to serve.

LOVELY LUNCHES

CHEDDAR AND MUSHROOM OMELETTE FOR ONE

Serves 1

Preparation time: 5 minutes

Cooking time: 10 minutes

The omelette contains 3g carbohydrate; 251 calories; 2.5g sugars; 16.5g fat; 0.7g salt; and 2 portions of vegetables.

Ingredients:

2 eggs

Pinch of white pepper

1 tsp sunflower oil

150g mushrooms, sliced

1 spring onion, chopped

10g reduced-fat Cheddar cheese

Method:

1. Break the eggs into a bowl, add the pepper and beat with a fork. Set aside.

2. Heat the oil in a frying pan and cook the mushrooms and spring onion for 5 minutes on a medium heat, stirring regularly until soft.

3. Stir the eggs into the mushrooms and spring onion, then cook gently for 3 minutes. Use a spatula to ease the omelette from the sides of the frying pan.

4. When the omelette is cooked, sprinkle the cheese on top and slide it out onto a plate, folding it in half so that the cheese is in the middle.

GLUTEN-FREE VEGGIE PIZZA

Serves 2

Preparation time: 30 minutes

Cooking time: 30 minutes

1 serving (half pizza) contains 18g carbohydrate; 382 calories; 34.8g sugars; 18.1g fat; 0.5g salt; and 3 portions of vegetables.

Ingredients:

1 cauliflower

1 tsp sunflower oil

75g red onion, thinly sliced

1 red pepper (optional), cored and chopped

150g courgette, diced

2 tomatoes, chopped

2 garlic cloves, crushed

1 heaped tsp dried oregano

1 egg, beaten

25g Parmesan cheese, finely grated

80g reduced-fat mozzarella cheese, thinly sliced

6–8 basil leaves, torn

½ tsp chilli flakes (optional)

Method:

1. Pre-heat the oven to 180°C/Gas mark 4. Remove the stalks from the cauliflower and break into florets. Hand grate or blitz the florets in a food processor.

2. Put the cauliflower in a bowl and cover with cling film, piercing the film a few times. Cook in a microwave on full power (800 watts) for 4–5 minutes, or steam it for 2 minutes, until soft. Allow to cool.

3. Once the cauliflower is completely cool, place it onto a clean tea towel and press it firmly to remove any excess water. Set aside.

4. Make the pizza topping: heat the oil in a frying pan and cook the onion, red pepper and courgette over a medium heat for 4–5 minutes until the onion is starting to brown. Add the tomatoes, garlic and oregano and cook for another 2 minutes. Mix well and set aside.

5. Add the cauliflower to a bowl with the egg and Parmesan and mix well.

6. Line a round baking tray or pizza sheet – 25cm in diameter – with non-stick baking paper and spread the cauliflower mixture to the thickness of 0.75cm onto it. Bake for 15 minutes. Remove from oven and add toppings. Bake for a further 10 minutes before removing from the oven. Add torn bay leaves and sprinkle with chilli flakes – if using.

ONION SOUP WITH POTATO WEDGES

Serves 4

Preparation time: 15 minutes

Cooking time: 50 minutes

Each serving contains 54.8g carbohydrate; 287 calories; 23g sugars;
5.8g fat; 0.9g salt; and 4 portions of vegetables.

Ingredients:

3 tsp sunflower oil

1kg onions, finely chopped

400g sweet potato, cut into wedges, skin on

1 low-salt vegetable stock cube dissolved in 800ml boiling water

4 slices of pre-cut wholemeal bread

20g reduced-fat mature Cheddar cheese, grated

1 tbsp parsley, finely chopped, plus extra to serve

1 tsp low-salt soy sauce

Good pinch of white pepper

Method:

1. Pre-heat the oven to 190°C/Gas mark 5. Add 2 tsp of the oil to a sauce-pan, then add the onions and cook over a very low heat for 30–40 minutes, stirring regularly so the onions caramelise.

2. Meanwhile, pour the remaining oil onto a baking sheet. Add the sweet potatoes and move them around to coat. Bake in oven for 30–40 minutes, until lightly browned.

3. While the wedges are cooking, add the stock to the onions, bring to the boil and simmer for 5 minutes.

4. Meanwhile make the cheesy croutons: cut each slice of bread in half and grill, then turn over and top each piece with Cheddar cheese and grill again, until the cheese melts and browns. Alternatively, you can

put the cheese-topped bread on a baking tray and cook it in the oven for 5–10 minutes.

5. Stir the parsley, soy sauce and pepper into the soup, then divide the soup equally into four bowls. Serve with cheesy croutons and a sprinkling of fresh parsley on top, and with the potato wedges on the side.

CHARGRILLED CHICKEN SALAD

Serves 4

Preparation time: 10 minutes

Cooking time: 20 minutes

Each serving contains 37.1g carbohydrate; 350 calories; 4.8g sugars; 11.5g fat; and 1.4g salt.

Ingredients:

For the dressing

30g Parmesan cheese, finely grated

2 tsp low-fat yoghurt

1 tbsp extra-virgin olive oil

1 tbsp Dijon mustard

Juice of ¼ lemon

1 tsp Worcestershire sauce

Pinch of white pepper

For the salad

2 skinless and boneless chicken breasts, sliced in half horizontally

1 tsp olive oil

80g little gem lettuce, leaves separated

For the croutons

1 garlic clove, crushed

½ tbsp olive oil

Pinch of black pepper

10cm length of baguette or ciabatta bread, cubed

10g Parmesan cheese shavings, to top

Method:

1. Pre-heat the oven to 180°C/Gas mark 4. Mix all of the dressing ingredients together and set aside to infuse.

2. To begin the salad, rub the thin chicken breasts in a little oil, then cook on a hot griddle pan for 2–3 minutes each side, or until thoroughly cooked through, then cut into strips.

3. To make the croutons, add the garlic and olive oil to a bowl and crush together with the back of a spoon. Add the black pepper, mix well and coat the insides of the bowl with the mixture.

4. Add the bread cubes and mix to coat in the oil. Spread the cubes on to a baking tray and bake in the oven for around 8–10 minutes, turning with a spatula so they don't burn, until browned.

5. To assemble the salad, layer the lettuce in a shallow bowl, saving the smaller leaves until last so you create concentric circles. Drizzle with the dressing, sprinkle with the croutons and chicken, and top with Parmesan shavings.

CREAMY BACON AND LEEK PASTA

Serves 2

Preparation time: 10 minutes

Cooking time: 12 minutes

Each serving contains 71.6g carbohydrate; 472 calories; 8.3g sugars;
10.4g fat; 1.8g salt; and 1 portion of vegetables.

Ingredients:

175g dried pasta shapes

2 rashers of lean back bacon, chopped

1 leek (about 150g), finely chopped

1 tsp chopped rosemary

1 small carton of natural yoghurt

1 tbsp sundried tomato paste

Freshly ground black pepper, to taste

A little grated Parmesan, to top

Salad vegetables, to serve

Method:

1. Cook the pasta according to the pack instructions, then drain and set aside.

2. Meanwhile, place the bacon into a frying pan and dry-fry for 2 minutes. Add the leeks and rosemary and fry for a further 3–4 minutes, until the leeks are cooked.

3. Mix together the yoghurt and sundried tomato paste and stir into the cooked pasta, adding the bacon, leeks, rosemary and black pepper to taste. Sprinkle a little Parmesan cheese on the top and serve with plenty of salad vegetables.

MOUTH-WATERING MAIN MEALS

GORGEOUS GOULASH

Serves 2

Preparation time: 15 minutes

Cooking time: 3 hours 5 minutes

One serving contains 36.6g carbohydrate; 370 calories; 12.7g sugars;
8.7g fat; 1.7g salt; and 2$^1/_3$ portions of vegetables.

Ingredients:

250g diced, lean braising steak

250g new potatoes

2 tsp seasoned plain flour (use black pepper and a salt substitute to season)

1 tsp sunflower oil

1 onion, chopped

½ red pepper, chopped

1 garlic clove, crushed

1 tsp paprika

200g chopped tomatoes

1 tsp tomato purée

150ml beef stock

Method:

1. Preheat the oven to 180°C/Gas mark 4.

2. Toss the steak in the seasoned flour. Heat the oil in a flameproof casserole dish, add the steak and fry for 2–3 minutes until brown all over.

3. Add the remaining ingredients and bring to the boil, then put the lid on the casserole dish and place in the oven for 3 hours, or until the meat is tender.

4. Serve with plenty of vegetables.

CHEESY SPINACH CANNELLONI

Serves 6

Preparation time: 5 minutes

Cooking time: 25 minutes

Each serving contains 20g carbohydrate; 160 calories; 4.8g fat;

5.5g sugar; 0.3g salt; and 1 portion of vegetables.

Ingredients:

1 tsp sunflower oil

1 large onion, finely chopped

1 leek, finely chopped

3 garlic cloves, crushed

250g frozen leaf spinach

150g ricotta cheese

½ tsp nutmeg

400g tin chopped tomatoes

1 tbsp oregano

1 tbsp tomato purée

A generous grind of black pepper

120g dried (no pre-cook) cannelloni pasta

25g mozzarella cheese, thinly sliced

Method:

1. Pre-heat the oven to 180°C/Gas mark 4.

2. Add the oil to a saucepan and cook the onion and leek for 5–8 minutes. Mix in the garlic and cook together for another couple of minutes, then remove from the heat.

3. Add the spinach, ricotta cheese and nutmeg to the pan and mix well.

4. Put the tomatoes in a bowl and add the oregano, tomato purée and black pepper. Mix together to make the sauce.

5. Stuff the spinach and ricotta mixture into the cannelloni. Put half the

tomato sauce in an ovenproof dish. Place the stuffed cannelloni on top and add the remaining sauce. Top with mozzarella and bake for 15 minutes until golden and bubbling.

ZINGY SALMON FILLETS

Serves 6

Preparation time: 10 minutes

Cooking time: 8 minutes

Each serving of marinated salmon contains 2.7g carbohydrate;
246 calories; 25g sugars; 15g fat; and 1.1g salt.

Ingredients:

6 skinless, boneless salmon fillets (about 125g each)

For the marinade

2 tbsp soy sauce

2 tsp sesame oil

A pinch of chilli flakes

1 tsp ginger, grated

1 tbsp chopped coriander, to garnish

4 spring onions, sliced, to garnish

Method:

1. Place the marinade ingredients into a non-metallic bowl and stir well.

2. Add the salmon fillets and coat in the marinade. Set aside for at least 5 minutes (longer for a stronger flavour) to allow the flavours to infuse.

3. Cook the marinated salmon fillets for 3–4 minutes in a pan on a medium heat, then add any remaining marinade, turning the salmon over to cook the other side for 3–4 minutes. (You may need to do this in batches.) Scatter over the coriander and spring onions before serving.

BUBBLE AND SQUEAK WITH POACHED EGGS

Serves 3

Preparation time: 15 minutes

Cooking time: 30 minutes

Each portion contains 31.2g carbohydrate; 325 calories;
8.7g sugars; 15.9g fat; 0.6g salt; and 1½ portions of vegetables.

Ingredients:

350g potatoes, peeled and cubed

1 large parsnip, peeled and cubed

4 tbsp skimmed milk

25g low-fat spread

1 tsp sunflower oil

1 small onion, chopped

1 large carrot, peeled and grated

100g green cabbage, finely shredded

3 medium eggs

Salt substitute and freshly ground black pepper

Method:

1. Cook the potatoes and parsnips together in boiling water for 12–15 minutes, or until soft. Drain and mash with the milk and low-fat spread. Season well.

2. Heat the oil in a medium frying pan. Add the onion, carrot and cabbage and fry for 5 minutes until cooked through.

3. Add the vegetables to the mashed potato and parsnip and form 3 equally sized patties. Fry each patty in a frying pan over a medium heat until brown on both sides.

4. Poach the eggs in boiling water and place one on top of each bubble and squeak patty, season and serve.

SWEET POTATO FISH PIE

Serves 6

Preparation time: 10 minutes

Cooking time: 45–55 minutes

Each serving contains 36.9g carbohydrate; 339 calories; 12.8g sugars;
8.4g fat; 0.9g salt; and 2 portions of vegetables.

Ingredients:

1kg sweet potatoes, peeled and chopped

1 tsp sunflower oil

2 leeks, halved lengthways, then sliced

1 heaped tsp plain flour

1 fish stock cube

400ml skimmed milk

Good pinch of white pepper

25g parsley, plus extra to garnish

1 heaped tsp paprika

300g skinless, boneless pollack, cut into cubes

300g skinless, boneless salmon, cut into cubes

Pinch of black pepper, to serve

Method:

1. Pre-heat the oven to 180°C/Gas mark 4. Cook the sweet potatoes in a pan of boiling water for 15–20 minutes until soft, then drain.

2. Meanwhile, heat the oil in a saucepan and fry the leeks, stirring regularly until soft, about 7 minutes.

3. Sprinkle the flour over the leeks and crumble the stock cube over. Mix well for a minute to coat the leeks.

4. Slowly stir in 100ml of the milk, until the leeks are coated in a thick paste, then gradually add in the remaining milk, stirring constantly until the mixture comes to the boil. Stir in the white pepper and parsley and remove the pan from the heat.

5. Mash the sweet potatoes until smooth and stir in the paprika.

6. Add the leek sauce to an oven-proof dish and arrange the fish so that it's evenly distributed over the top. Top with the sweet potato and bake for 25–35 minutes, until the sauce starts to bubble through the sweet potato. Sprinkle with parsley and black pepper.

DELIGHTFUL DESSERTS

APPLE PUDDING

Serves 4

Preparation time: 10 minutes

Cooking time: 20 minutes

Each serving contains 27.6g carbohydrate;

162 calories; 7.4g sugar; 3.2g fat; 0.5g salt; and 1 portion of fruit.

Ingredients:

3 unpeeled apples, cored and grated

200ml apple juice, plus extra if required

1 tbsp blackstrap molasses

1 tsp cinnamon

4–5 slices of wholemeal bread, crusts removed

1 egg yolk, lightly beaten

Low-fat yoghurt or crème fraîche, to serve (optional)

Method:

1. Pre-heat the oven to 180°C/Gas mark 4. Put the apple in a saucepan with 100ml of the apple juice and place over a low heat. Simmer for 4–5 minutes, until the apples have softened. Leaving the juice in the pan, place the apple in a bowl and set aside.

2. Add the molasses and cinnamon to the pan with the remaining 100ml of apple juice. Allow the molasses to melt gently, adding a little more juice if needed to make about 100ml of syrup. Allow to cool.

3. Grease a small pudding basin with a little sunflower oil and line the basin with the bread – keeping some to seal the top. Pour the syrup into the basin, reserving some for soaking the bread that will go on top.

4. Stir the egg yolk into the cooked apple and put the mixture into the pudding basin. Top with the remaining bread and pour on the last of the syrup.

5. Bake for 15 minutes and check the pudding – if the top is very brown at the edges, place a piece of foil over the top. Then, bake for a further 5 minutes.

6. Allow the pudding to stand for a couple of minutes before loosening with a knife around the edge of the basin. Carefully turn out the apple pudding onto a serving plate. Serve with a little low-fat plain yoghurt or low-fat crème fraîche, if you wish.

FRUITY ICE CREAM

Serves 4

Preparation time: 15 minutes, plus 2½ hours for freezing

Cooking time: 15 minutes

Each serving contains 28.9g carbohydrate; 312 calories; 31.4g sugar;

8.1g fat; 0.2g salt; and 1 portion of fruit.

Ingredients:

600ml unsweetened soya milk

Few drops of vanilla extract

1 tbsp cornflour

4 egg yolks

2 tbsp confectioner's sugar

300g tinned blackcurrants in unsweetened, natural juice, drained

200g frozen raspberries

Method:

1. Place the milk and vanilla extract into a medium-sized saucepan and bring to the boil.

2. In a bowl, whisk together the cornflour, egg yolks and confectioner's sugar.

3. Pour the milk over the cornflour mixture and stir in. Return mixture to saucepan and place over a low heat until the mixture thickens. Do not boil, otherwise the mixture will curdle. Remove from the heat.

4. Cool the mixture, then stir in the blackcurrants and raspberries.

5. Transfer to a freezer-proof container.

6. Freeze the ice-cream mixture for 15 minutes, then remove from freezer and break up the ice crystals with a fork. Re-freeze for a further 1 hour, then take it out of the freezer and break up the ice crystals with a fork again. Place the ice cream back in freezer for at least another 1 hour and 15 minutes. Remove from the freezer and allow to stand for 10 minutes before serving.

PARADISE RICE PUDDING

Serves 4

Preparation time: 3 minutes

Cooking time: 30 minutes

Each serving contains 32g carbohydrate; 179 calories; 6g sugars;

4g fat; 0.3g salt.

Ingredients:

100g Basmati rice

400ml can reduced-fat coconut milk

300ml soya milk

25g caster sugar or 2 dessert spoons of granulated artificial sweetener

Few drops of vanilla extract

1 tbsp toasted coconut

Method:

1. Place all the ingredients except the toasted coconut into a small saucepan. Place over a low heat and simmer very gently for 20–30 minutes until the rice is tender.

2. Transfer to a serving dish, top with toasted coconut and serve.

INDULGENT BLUEBERRY AND LEMON CHEESECAKE

Serves 1

Preparation time: 5 minutes

Serving contains 33.9g carbohydrate; 279 calories; 19g sugars;
11.5g fat; 1.1g salt; and 1 portion of fruit.

Ingredients:

Finely grated zest of ½ a lemon, plus 1 tsp lemon juice

1 heaped tsp lemon curd

1 heaped tsp reduced-fat cream cheese (about 60g)

75g blueberries, plus extra to garnish

2 oat cakes, crushed

Method:

1. Combine the lemon zest, lemon curd and cream cheese in a bowl.

2. Gently crush half the blueberries with a fork and add the lemon juice.

3. Add the remaining blueberries to the cream cheese mixture.

4. Place the crushed blueberries at the bottom of a serving glass. Top with the lemony cheese mixture and sprinkle with crushed oat cake. Garnish with the remaining blueberries.

FRUITY TRIFLE

Serves 10

Preparation time: 25 minutes, plus 2 hours cooling

Cooking time: 15 minutes

Each serving contains 9g carbohydrate; 120 calories; 4.1g sugars;
6.8g fat; 0.2g salt; and 1 portion of fruit.

Ingredients:

For the sponge

40g wholemeal flour

½ tsp baking powder

5 tsp granulated sugar substitute

2 tbsp light olive oil, plus a little extra for greasing

1 small egg, beaten

1 tsp of vanilla extract

For the custard

250ml skimmed milk

20g cornflour

1 tsp vanilla extract

5 tsp granulated sweetener

2 tsp semi-skimmed milk

For the jelly

23g sachet of sugar-free strawberry jelly crystals

300g frozen mixed berries

For the topping

200g low-fat Greek yoghurt

200g half-fat crème fraîche

10g toasted flaked almonds

Grated zest of 1 lemon

Method:

1. To make the sponge: in a bowl, mix together the flour, baking powder and sweetener. Add the 2 tablespoons of oil, the egg and the vanilla extract and mix thoroughly until smooth.

2. Add 50ml of water and beat. Lightly oil a 570ml microwave-proof bowl and pour in the mixture.

3. Microwave on full power (800 watts) for 2 minutes and 20 seconds, then allow to cool.

4. To make the custard, put the milk in a saucepan and bring to the boil.

5. Meanwhile, put the cornflour, vanilla extract, sweetener and semi-skimmed milk in a cup and mix well until smooth.

6. Once the milk is about to boil, stir in the cornflour mixture, stirring continuously with a wooden spoon and bring to boiling point, stirring until thickened. Remove from the heat and leave to cool.

7. To assemble, break the sponge into pieces and scatter on the bottom of a glass bowl.

8. Make the jelly according to the packet instructions, but use 10 per cent less water than stated. Set aside and allow to cool for 10 minutes.

9. Scatter the frozen berries on top of the sponge, then pour the jelly over the fruit and sponge and place in the fridge for 30 minutes to set.

10. Spread the custard over the jelly and return the trifle to the fridge for 30 minutes. Cover with cling film and refrigerate until you're ready to serve (overnight if you wish).

11. To finish the trifle, mix the yoghurt and the crème fraîche together and use to top the custard, then scatter with almonds and lemon zest.

TASTY TREATS

FABULOUS FRUIT CAKE

(This also makes an excellent Christmas cake)

Serves 12

Preparation time: 20 minutes

Cooking time: 1½ hours

Each serving contains 24.8g carbohydrate; 197 calories; 4.3g sugars; 8.4g fat; 0.2g salt; and 1 portion of fruit.

Ingredients:

75g sultanas

100g raisins

250g candied peel

100ml boiling water

1 banana (about 100g), mashed

2 eggs, beaten

75ml sunflower oil

1 courgette (about 200g), grated

1 apple (about 100g), grated

1 carrot (about 80g), finely grated

150g wholemeal flour

1 tsp baking powder

3 tsp mixed spice

6 glacé cherries

20g whole blanched almonds

Method:

1. Pre-heat the oven to 170°C/Gas mark 3. Add the sultanas, raisins and peel to a bowl. Cover with the boiling water and set aside.

2. Mix together the mashed banana, eggs and oil in a large bowl and beat well to combine.

3. Mix the courgette, apple and carrot into the banana, then stir in the flour, baking powder and mixed spice. Next, add the rehydrated dried fruit, plus the soaking water.

4. Stir to combine thoroughly and put the mixture into a 20cm cake tin lined with baking parchment. Top the mixture with cherries and almonds, cover with foil and bake for 1½ hours. Remove the foil 15–20 minutes before the end of the cooking time, then bake uncovered for the remainder of the time, until the top is browned and a knife or skewer inserted into the centre of the cake comes out clean. Leave to cool in the tin for 10 minutes, then turn out onto a wire rack, invert so that the cherries are on the top again and leave to cool completely.

CHEESY SCONES

Makes 10

Preparation time: 15 minutes

Cooking time: 15 minutes

Each scone contains 14.7g carbohydrate; 113 calories; 0.7g sugars;
3.9g fat; 0.2g salt; and a quarter of a portion of vegetables.

Ingredients:

200g wholemeal flour

1 tsp baking powder

Pinch of white pepper

75g frozen spinach, defrosted with excess water removed to give 50g

4 spring onions, chopped finely

50g low-fat mature Cheddar cheese, grated

2 tbsp sunflower oil

75ml skimmed milk

½ tsp paprika (optional)

Method:

1. Pre-heat the oven to 180°C/Gas mark 4, then place a large baking tray in the oven.

2. Mix the flour, baking powder and pepper together, add the spinach and spring onions, then sprinkle the grated cheese, reserving 2 tsp of cheese for later, into the mixture to distribute it evenly.

3. Make a well in the centre of the mixture and pour in the oil and half the milk. Mix together. Reserve 1 tbsp of milk for glazing, then add the remaining milk little by little, until you have a soft but firm dough.

4. Lightly flour the work surface and gently roll out the dough until 2cm thick. Cut out the scones with a medium-sized round cutter and place on the hot oven tray. Pull together any scraps of dough and roll out again to get an extra couple of scones.

5. Glaze the tops of the scones with the reserved milk and sprinkle with the reserved cheese, and some paprika if you wish.

6. Bake for 12–15 minutes, until golden brown. Serve warm.

BLACKBERRY AND APPLE DELIGHT

Makes 12 slices

Preparation time: 10 minutes

Cooking time: 40 minutes

Each slice contains 17.7g carbohydrate; 156 calories; 7.3g sugars;
7.5g fat; 0.1g salt; and 1 portion of fruit.

Ingredients:

100ml sunflower oil

2 apples, cored and grated (skin on)

2 medium eggs

1 tsp vanilla extract

75g caster sugar or 6 dessert spoons of granulated sweetener

150g wholemeal flour

1 tsp baking powder

150g blackberries

Method:

1. Pre-heat the oven to 180°C/Gas mark 4. Use 1 tsp of the oil to grease a 450g loaf tin.

2. Put the grated apple into a bowl, then add the eggs, vanilla extract, sugar substitute and oil and beat together.

3. Add the flour and baking powder and mix well. Fold in the blackberries.

4. Pour the mixture into the prepared loaf tin and bake for 25 minutes until firm and golden and a knife or skewer inserted into the centre comes out clean. Cover with foil after 20 minutes if it's starting to brown too much.

CHERRY AND CHOCOLATE DELIGHT

Serves 4

Preparation time: 20 minutes

Cooking time: 20 minutes

Each serving contains 19g carbohydrate; 114 calories; 8g sugars; 2.2g fat;
0.1g salt; and half a portion of fruit.

Ingredients:

225g fresh cherries, halved and destoned, reserving 4 whole cherries for
decoration

2 tbsp granulated sugar substitute

1 tsp cornflour mixed to a paste with 1 tsp water

100g quark or low-fat soft cheese

2 tbsp skimmed milk

½ tsp vanilla extract

For the chocolate sauce

25g dark chocolate, broken into pieces

1 heaped tsp unsweetened cocoa powder

½ tsp cornflour mixed to a paste with ½ tsp water

1 tsp blackstrap molasses

Method:

1. Put the halved cherries into a saucepan with 50ml of water. Add
    1 teaspoon of the artificial sweetener and simmer for 30 minutes,
    until the cherries are soft, then leave on the heat and stir in the
    cornflour paste. Remove from the heat, stirring to prevent a skin
    forming.

2. In a bowl, beat the low-fat soft cheese, skimmed milk, vanilla extract
    and remaining sweetener together until smooth. Set aside.

3. For the chocolate sauce: put the dark chocolate pieces into a small
    saucepan and add the unsweetened cocoa powder, the cornflour paste

and the molasses. Place over a moderate heat, stirring constantly until smooth. Cool, stirring to prevent a skin forming.

4. Spoon the soft cheese mixture into 4 small serving glasses, putting cherries in first, pouring chocolate sauce over or creating layers, according to your own preference. Top each serving with a whole cherry, chill and serve.

SPICY GINGER BISCUITS

Makes 24

Preparation time: 10 minutes

Cooking time: 25 minutes

Each biscuit contains 7.1g carbohydrate; 56 calories; 1.3g sugars;
2.0g fat; 0.1g salt.

Ingredients:

50ml sunflower oil

10g blackstrap molasses

100ml skimmed milk

100g wholemeal flour

1 tsp baking powder

3 tsp powdered ginger

1 tsp mixed spice

8 tsp granulated sugar substitute

1 egg, beaten

1 ripe banana, mashed

Method:

1. Pre-heat the oven to 150°C/Gas mark 2. Place the oil, molasses and milk in a saucepan and heat gently for 2 minutes.

2. Meanwhile, in a bowl, mix together the flour, baking powder, ginger, mixed spice and sweetener. Beat together the egg and mashed banana and add to the bowl with the flour mixture.

3. Line a 30cm baking tray with baking parchment. Gently stir the oil and molasses mixture into the flour mixture and pour into the lined tin (the biscuit will be about 1cm thick). Bake in the centre of the oven for 1 hour, or until the centre of the mixture is firm to the touch.

4. Remove from the oven and leave the biscuit to cool in the tin for 15–20 minutes. Transfer to a chopping board and cut into individual squares.

Helpful Hints and Tips

'You need to know where you can get some help to deal with it all.'

There are things you can do to allow other people to share your diabetes self-care with you – it helps them to feel valued, useful and part of things and it helps you manage your condition:

- You should participate in agreeing your self-care goals and treatment plan with your diabetes team and take the advice you're given seriously.
- Tell your employer you have diabetes and make sure the people you work with know how to treat a hypo.
- Teach your friends and relatives how to recognise a hypo – list the symptoms and pass it round – and how they should react.
- Keep your BG as near-normal as you can – between 5.0 and 7.0 mmol/L – to avoid the onset of complications. Make sure you have an annual eye examination, blood, urine and nerve tests, and regular foot checks. It is your responsibility to make sure these are done.
- Exercise regularly with a friend or relative – walk the dog together or go swimming with someone. Having a commitment to meet up will help you do planned exercise and not put it off.
- Make sure you have the contact details for a direct-access chiropodist if you suddenly develop a problem with your feet and you need to refer yourself to someone who can help as soon as possible. You can get these details from your GP surgery.
- Tell your family what you should be eating so they can help prepare the right foods and you can find restaurants together that serve healthy options rather than high-fat, high-calorie meals. If other people are also eating healthy options, you won't feel like you're missing out.

- Once you've come to terms with your diagnosis and have accepted that you have diabetes, you should receive a course of diabetes education as this is vital for you to manage your condition properly. If you haven't received this already, ask your diabetes team or your GP for information.
- Make sure you know how your diabetes medication works, how long it works for, and when it might not work properly – such as if it's taken with other medications.
- Work with a dietician so you can still enjoy your favourite foods. The dietician in your diabetes team wants to help make having diabetes as easy as possible for you so it fits into your lifestyle as painlessly as possible.
- Make sure you are up to date with advances in diabetes care as things are changing all the time and new developments become reality. You can discuss this with your diabetes team and/or GP. Remember – if you don't ask, you don't get!

Useful contacts

DIABETES UK
Tel: 0207 424 1000 (language line available)
Minicom: 0207 462 2757
Website: www.diabetes.org.uk
Email: info@diabetes.org.uk

THE DIABETES FEDERATION OF IRELAND
Aims to help people with diabetes and their families
www.diabetesireland.ie

DIABETES IN SCOTLAND
Provides information about diabetes and its treatment.
www.diabetesinscotland.org.uk

HEALTH OF WALES INFORMATION SERVICE – HOWIS

Provides health and lifestyle information for the population of Wales.

www.wales.nhs.uk

THE AMERICAN DIABETES ASSOCIATION

Tel: 800-342-2383

www.diabetes.org

DOSE ADJUSTMENT FOR NORMAL EATING – DAFNE

www.dafne.uk.com

ROYAL NATIONAL INSTITUTE FOR THE BLIND – RNIB

www.rnib.org.uk

DESMOND – Type 2 DIABETES WEBSITE

Tel: 0116 258 5881

Email: desmondweb@uhl-tr.nhs.uk

Website: www.desmond-project.org.uk

NATIONAL SERVICE FRAMEWORK – NSF – FOR DIABETES

This Department of Health document describes the standard of diabetes care you should receive.

www.doh.gov.uk/nsf/diabetes

CARBOHYDRATE EXCHANGE WEBSITE

This website shows you the carbohydrate content of any food you want to find out about.

www.eatright.org/cps/rde/xchg/ada/hs.xsl/nutrition_13961_ENU_HTML.htm

DIABETIC RETINOPATHY WEBSITE

Provides information about retinopathy prevention, treatment and research.

www.diabeticretinopathy.org.uk

FEET FOR LIFE
The Society of Chiropodists and Podiatrists website to help with all foot problems.
www.feetforlife.org

NHS DIRECT ONLINE
NHS Direct Online provides health advice and information.
www.nhsdirect.nhs.uk

NETDOCTOR.CO.UK
The UK's leading health website written by doctors and health professionals.
www.netdoctor.co.uk/diabetes/index.shtml

BBC HEALTH DIABETES GUIDE
This guide explains diabetes, its symptoms, causes and treatments.
www.bbc.co.uk/health/diabetes

PREGNANCY AND DIABETES
A section on the Diabetes UK website providing useful advice and information.
www.diabetes.org.uk/pregnancy

THE DIABETES TRAVEL INFORMATION WEBSITE
Provides information to help you anticipate any diabetes-related issues before your journey. www.diabetes-travel.co.uk

MEDIC ALERT
Medic Alert is a charity providing inscribed jewellery with alerts to health conditions and allergies.
www.medicalert.co.uk

DIABETES INSIGHT
Diabetes Insight provides information and a discussion forum about the condition.
www.diabetes-insight.info

JUVENILE DIABETES RESEARCH FOUNDATION – JDRF
JDRF supports Type 1 diabetes in children and young adults
www.jdrf.org

CHILDREN WITH DIABETES
Gives advice about meal planning and nutrition, as well as recipes.
www.childrenwithdiabetes.com

DIABETES RESEARCH & WELLNESS FOUNDATION – DRWF
Organisation aiming to help people with diabetes to live a healthy life.
www.diabeteswellnessnet.org.uk

THE NATIONAL INSTITUTE FOR HEALTH AND CARE EXCELLENCE
– NICE
Part of the NHS, providing guidance on medications and best practice.
www.NICE.org.uk
The information is also available in Welsh and in large print for the visually
impaired.

THE INSULIN PUMP THERAPY GROUP – INPUT
Helps people access technology to improve their BG control.
Tel: 0800 228 9977
Email: info@inputdiabetes.org.uk Website: www.inputdiabetes.org.uk

MIND
Charity supporting people with mental health issues.
www.mind.com

GOOD MENTAL HEALTH MATTERS.COM
Provides support and information for emotional, psychological and social
wellbeing.
goodmentalhealthmatters.com

DIABETIC EXERCISE AND SPORTS ASSOCIATION
A website where you can find out the right kind of exercise for you.
www.diabetes-exercise.org

DISABILITY RIGHTS COMMISSION
Website: www.drc-gb.org
Email enquiries: ddahelp@stra.sitel.co.uk

THE ASIAN COOKERY CLUB
Provides information about nutrition and recipes.
www.lutonpct.nhs.uk/cookclub.htm

Further reading

Quick and Easy Cooking for Diabetes
by Jenny Bryan, published by Hodder Wayland

Real Food for Diabetics
by Molly Perham, published by Foulsham

Diabetes Diet Book: Type 2
by Calvin Ezrin, published by Contemporary Books Inc.

Prevent & Cure Diabetes: Delicious Diets, Not Dangerous Drugs
by Sarah Mayhill & Craig Robinson, published by Hammersmith Health Books

Sugarless, Not Flavourless: Delicious Sugar-Free Sweets & Treats That Taste Like the Real Thing
by Catherine Singh, published by CreateSpace Independent Publishing

Say No to Diabetes
by Patrick Holford, published by Piatkus

The 8-Week Blood Sugar Diet Recipe Book: 150 Simple, Delicious Recipes to Keep Your Blood Sugar Levels in Check
by Claire Bailey & Sarah Schenker, published by Short Books

Nutritional Medicine
by Dr Stephen Davies & Dr Alan Stewart, published by Pan Books

The Better Pregnancy Diet
by Patrick & Liz Holford, published by ION Press

How to Boost Your Immune System
by Christopher Scarfe, published by ION Press

The GI Diet Pocket Guide
by Rick Gallop, published by Virgin Books

Glossary of Terms

Acanthosis nigricans – a condition associated with Type 2 diabetes where velvety areas of skin develop with increased pigmentation on the back of the neck and armpits. It shows a strong racial disposition and is common in Indian, Hispanic and black populations.

Addison's disease – a condition that affects the adrenal glands that sit on top of the kidneys. The condition can cause frequent and severe hypoglycaemia – low BG levels – because it affects hormones that maintain the amount of glucose in the blood.

Adrenaline – released by the adrenal glands in response to stress, increasing the rate of breathing, pushing up heart rate, and improving muscle performance in the *fight or flight response*.

Alpha-blockers – medications such as Doxazosin derivatives, used to treat high blood pressure.

Alpha Glucosidase Inhibitors – a group of glucose-reducing medications for the treatment of Type 2 diabetes including Acarbose (Precose) and Miglitol (Glyset).

Anaemia – iron deficiency.

Anorexia – a mental health disorder where there is an obsessive fear of gaining weight, resulting in severe dietary restriction.

Asthma – a condition characterised by breathlessness owing to generalised narrowing of the airways throughout the lungs. There are two different types of asthma in terms of the cause: extrinisic, where external factors – allergens – such as smoke, pollen, dust, etc. trigger an attack, and intrinsic, where there is no apparent external cause.

Atherosclerosis – degenerative disease of the arteries associated with fatty deposits on the inner walls, leading to reduced blood flow.

Auto-immune attack – the body's defence mechanism. Type 1 diabetes is an auto-immune disease where the body attacks its own insulin-producing cells in the pancreas.

Auto-immune conditions – conditions caused by auto-immune attack: asthma, Type 1 diabetes, coeliac disease and psoriasis are all examples.

Auto-immune syndrome – a condition resulting in a high concentration of insulin in the blood, despite low BG levels.

Autonomic neuropathy – damage to the autonomic nerves controlling involuntary functions such as digestion and cardiac functions.

Basal rate – the rate of background insulin delivered by an insulin pump so a person can keep their BG levels within normal limits without eating or going too high or low.

Bendrofluozide – medication that reduces blood pressure but can increase BG levels.

Beta-carotene – the vegetable form of vitamin A.

Biguanides – a group of glucose-reducing medications for the treatment of Type 2 diabetes including Metformin – Glucophage; Metformin liquid – Riomet; Metformin extended release – Glucophage XR; Foramet – Glumetza.

Bile Acid Sequestrants – a group of glucose-reducing medications for the treatment of Type 2 diabetes including Colesevelam – Welchol.

Blood glucose level – the amount of glucose present in the blood. This varies according to the site where it is measured – blood from the fingertips gives the most up-to-date reading.

Blood plasma – the liquid part of the blood.

BMI – Body Mass Index: 20–20.9 = normal; 25–29.9 = overweight; 30 and above = obese.

Bolus – a dosage of insulin for meals or high BG levels.

Brittle diabetes – Type 1 diabetes that is very difficult to control, with erratic swings in BG from high to low.

Bulimia – a mental health disorder characterised by binge eating, then vomiting and/or laxative abuse.

Calorie – a unit of heat energy: the energy needed to raise the temperature of 1kg of water by 1°C.

Cannula – a small plastic tube that is inserted under the skin to deliver insulin in insulin pump therapy treatment.

Cataract – a chronic complication of diabetes manifesting as clouding of the lenses of the eyes, impairing vision.

Cardiac arrhythmia – an alteration in the normal heart rhythm.

Cardiomyopathy – a serious condition of the heart and circulatory system thought to stem from damage to the nerves controlling parts of the body not under conscious control, for example, the heartbeat.

Carpal Tunnel Syndrome – a chronic complication of diabetes where the tendons of the hand tighten and draw the fingers into a claw-like position.

CCG – County Commissioning Group, the local Health Authority in every county in the UK that decides on and pays for the funding of treatments such as insulin pump therapy and Continuous Glucose Monitoring to treat Type 1 diabetes.

CDNS – Children's Diabetes Nurse Specialist.

CGM – Continuous Glucose Monitoring – a piece of technology for use with insulin pump therapy where a plasma glucose sensor is inserted under the skin every six days and this is connected to a small transmitter that relays the glucose information to the pump for display. The user can then monitor high and low BG levels and act accordingly.

Charcot joints – also known as neuroarthropathy – a chronic complication of diabetes that refers to the degeneration of, for example, the joints of the foot owing to nerve damage, loss of sensation, and areas of pressure.

Cholesterol – blood fats.

Cimetidine – a medication prescribed for indigestion.

Coeliac disease – a systemic condition (having an effect on the whole body) that is a chronic auto-immune condition triggered by an intolerance to gluten – a protein found in cereal grains, such as wheat.

Combination Pills – a group of glucose-reducing medications for the treatment of Type 2 diabetes including Pioglitazone & Metformin; Actoplus Met; Glyburide & Metformin – Glucovance; Glipizide & Metformin – Metaglip; Sitagliptin & Metformin – Janumet; Saxagliptin & Metformin – Kombiglyze; Repaglinide & Metformin – Prandimet; Pioglitazone & Glimerpiride – Duetact.

Complications: acute – hypoglycaemia and diabetic ketoacidosis (DKA) are classed as acute complications of diabetes because they are short-term and can be reversed quickly.

Complications: chronic – chronic complications of diabetes appear over many years owing to high BG levels and can affect any part of the body. The main chronic complications are diabetic retinopathy – affecting the eyes; diabetic neuropathy – affecting the nerves; nephropathy – affecting the kidneys; coronary heart disease; and stroke – affecting the brain.

Condition specific – the knowledge and understanding your partner has about your diabetes and how it affects you.

Corticosteroids – medications that come as tablets, inhalers, injections or creams used to reduce inflammation.

Cortisol – a hormone released by the adrenal glands in response to stress, which raises BG levels, supresses the immune system and slows digestion.

DAFNE – Dose Adjustment For Normal Eating – a diabetes education course for people with Type 1.

Depression – symptoms must be categorised as distressing to the individual, or must cause a decline in social, occupational or other key functions to constitute a diagnosis of depression; symptoms that result from taking illicit drugs or prescription medication, or that arise from bereavement are not counted. Unfortunately, symptoms arising from the burden of diabetes self-care are also not recognised in making a diagnosis of depression, meaning that the mental and physical toll diabetes takes on the individual is often discounted.

DESMOND – Diabetes Education and Self-Management for Ongoing and Newly-Diagnosed – a diabetes education course for people with Type 2 diabetes.

Diabetes insipidus – a rare condition affecting the pituitary gland, which manifests as severe thirst and excessive urination that does not contain glucose.

Diabulimia – deliberately omitting or under-dosing on insulin to induce diabetic ketoacidosis and rapid weight loss.

Distal polyneuropathy – damage to many of the nerves in the hands and feet.

Diuretics – prescribed 'water' tablets that make you urinate more often.

DKA: see *ketoacidosis*.

DPP-4 Inhibitors – a group of glucose-reducing medications for the treatment of Type 2 diabetes including Sitagliptin – Januvia; Saxagliptin – Oxglyza; and Linaglyptin – Tradienta.

Dupuytren's disease – refers to a chronic complication seen in people with and without diabetes where the tendons of the wrists and hands tighten and the skin on the palms thickens.

DVLA – Driver and Vehicle Licensing Authority.

eAG – equivalent to HbA1c measurement in the USA.

Electrolytes – minerals like sodium and potassium, needed for nerve and muscle function and to help convert substances like protein into new cells.

Endorphins – hormones that promote a feeling of wellbeing.

Epinephrine – also known as adrenaline – a hormone that is also used as a medication.

Erectile dysfunction – inability to have or sustain an erection.

Exudates – a mass of cells and fluid that seeps out of a blood vessel or an organ, especially when there is inflammation.

Fair BG control – 7.0–8.0 mmol/L.

Fasting hypoglycaemia – a condition where BG levels are low owing to inadequate stores of glycogen – such as when dieting, or due to the slow conversion of glycogen into glucose when needed. The condition may also occur due to the consumption of alcohol, and breast or adrenal cancer.

Fibric acid derivatives – medications used to treat fat disorders.

Fight or flight response – a physical reaction to a perceived harmful event, attack or threat to survival where the options are to fight the threat, run from the threat, or freeze in the hope that the threat won't harm us or because we are paralysed with fear.

Flash glucose sensor – device measuring plasma glucose beneath the skin.

Folic acid – vitamin B9.

Foot ulcers – a situation where areas of pressure on the feet cannot be detected as pain so hard skin develops. Over time, this continued pressure on the hardened skin causes it to break down and soften until it grows mushy and comes away, leaving a deep hole, or ulcer, in the foot that becomes infected. If professional help is not sought for a diabetic foot ulcer, the hole enlarges and the blood supply dies off. At this stage, amputation is the only option – possibly the whole of the lower leg – to save the person's life.

Gastroparesis – delayed stomach emptying caused by damage to the autonomic nerves.

Gabapentin – also known as Neurontin – a medication that reduces nerve pain in neuropathy.

Gestational diabetes – develops in 2–4 per cent of women at around 28 weeks of pregnancy.

Ginkgo biloba – a tree bark traditionally eaten in China to improve blood flow to the arms, legs, fingers and toes. It is still used today and is also thought to improve memory.

Glaucoma – a condition where there is increased pressure within the eyeball, causing gradual loss of sight.

Glucagen hypo kit – a hormone injection that increases BG by slowing down involuntary muscle movement of the stomach and intestines. It is used to treat severe hypoglycaemia when the person is unconscious.

Glucose – a type of sugar.

Glucose intolerance – a term for conditions that increase BG, causing hyperglycaemia.

Glucose tolerance factor – a compound containing chromium that helps insulin to regulate BG levels.

Glucose tolerance test – when 75 grams of glucose is given by mouth, a BG result after two hours that is above 7.8 mmol/L (140.4 mg/dl American measurement), but below 11.1 mmol/L (199.8 mg/dl) is generally accepted as impaired glucose tolerance.

Glycaemic Index – the degree to which carbohydrates and starches raise BG relating to the speed that they are absorbed by the body.

Glycogen (glucose) – stored carbohydrate in the liver and body tissues.

Glycogen Storage Disease – a condition where the enzyme that breaks down stored glycogen into glucose is faulty, causing slow-release of glucose by the liver, resulting in hypoglycaemia.

Graves' disease – an enlarged and over-active thyroid gland.

Hashimoto's thyroiditis – a condition causing the thyroid gland to produce less thyroid hormone.

HbA1c – also known as haemoglobin A1c and glycosylated haemoglobin – measures the amount of glucose that sticks to the red blood cells over a three-month period before they are replaced.

Hereditary Fructose Disorder – a condition causing hypoglycaemia in children because the body can't metabolise natural fruit sugars.

Honeymoon period – can occur in children with Type 1 diabetes where the body's attack on the insulin-producing cells of the pancreas is not sufficient to wipe out all cells as soon as they are formed. When the honeymoon period ends and the pancreas stops producing insulin again in Type 1 diabetes – up to a period of 3 years – BG will begin to rise again.

Hydrocortisone – substances that reduce inflammation.

Hyperglycaemia – high BG levels caused by a lack of insulin.

Hyperostosis – a condition seen in people with Type 2 diabetes where the vertebrae of the spine fuse together.

Hypertension – high blood pressure.

Hypervitaminosis – a build-up of fat-soluble vitamins A, E and K in the body.

Hypoglycaemia – low BG caused by too much insulin, or strenuous exercise, or a lack of food, or because medication has reduced BG.

Hypoglycaemic unawareness – loss of awareness of the symptoms of low BG, such as tingling or sweating, or owing to autonomic nerve damage.

Hypostop – glucose gel, treatment for hypoglycaemia.

Hypothermia – a reduction in core body temperature to below 35°C.

Hypothyroidism – an under-active thyroid gland.

Impaired glucose tolerance – where the body is unable to deal with glucose because the action of insulin to bring down BG levels is impaired.

Infusion set – used with insulin pump therapy to deliver insulin via a small cannula placed under the skin and a thin plastic tube going from the cannula to the insulin pump.

Insulin – a hormone produced in the pancreas that controls the amount of glucose in the blood.

Insulin insensitivity – the ability of body cells to use insulin correctly to reduce BG levels.

Insulinoma – an insulin-producing tumour, usually benign.

Insulin pump therapy – also known as CSII: Continuous Subcutaneous Insulin Infusion – a piece of technology that delivers insulin in measured doses directly under the skin.

Insulin Resistance Syndrome – where glucose absorption by cells stimulated by insulin is reduced, increasing blood glucose levels and, in response, the amount of insulin that the body produces to cope with these increases.

Intermediate-acting insulin – NPH – a type of insulin used to treat Type 1 diabetes that covers the BG rise when rapid-acting insulin stops working. It is usually taken twice a day with rapid- or short-acting insulin, taking ninety minutes to four hours to reach the bloodstream where it works for up to twenty-four hours.

Irritable bowel syndrome – IBS – a common gut disorder with symptoms such as abdominal pain, bloating, diarrhoea and constipation. These symptoms come and go.

Islets of Langerhans – the insulin-producing cells of the pancreas.

Ketoacidosis – also known as DKA – breakdown of fats as an alternative source of energy to glucose, which can't be used when there's a lack of insulin.

Ketones – products from the breakdown of fats that build up in the blood and are excreted in the urine. Ketone bodies are acids that cause sickness and vomiting when there is high BG.

Kussmaul breathing – rapid breathing or panting that occurs during diabetic ketoacidosis as the body tries to excrete some of the acid build-up via the lungs. The breath smells like acetone – nail polish remover, or pear drops.

LGV – Large Goods Vehicle.

Long-acting insulin – used to reduce BG levels in the treatment of Type 1 diabetes and includes Lantus and Levemir that are usually combined with rapid- or short-acting insulin. It reaches the bloodstream from forty minutes to four hours after administering, where it works for up to twenty-four hours.

Macular degeneration – a condition where the central part of the retina at the back of the eye deteriorates. This is the leading cause of vision loss in people over the age of 60.

Macular oedema – fluid build-up causing loss of vision.

Meglitinides – a group of glucose-reducing medications for the treatment of Type 2 diabetes including Repagunide – Prandin; D-Phenylalanine derivatives; and Nanteglinide – Starlix.

Melatonin – a hormone produced by the pineal gland, the action of which supresses libido in accordance with the fight or flight response by reducing luteinising hormone and follicle stimulating hormone secretion by the anterior pituitary gland.

Metabolic syndrome – a group of associated conditions including coronary heart disease; high blood pressure; high levels of blood fats such as cholesterol; high levels of chemicals that prevent the breakdown of blood clots in the arteries and heart; and obesity.

Metformin – a medication used to treat Type 2 diabetes that lowers BG levels.

Metoclopramide – a medication used for gastroparesis (delayed stomach emptying) that increases muscle contraction in the digestive tract and speeds up the rate of stomach emptying.

Mmol/L – millimoles per litre.

Morbid obesity – a Body Mass Index of 45 and above.

Motor nerve damage – damage to the nerves that carry impulses to the muscles to make them move.

Multiple Daily Injections (MDI) – multiple daily injections or multiple dose insulin.

Necrobiosis lipoidica – a skin condition associated with diabetes where patches of reddish-brown skin form which can become thin and ulcerate.

Neuropathy – the term for nerve damage caused by long-term high BG levels in diabetes.

Nephropathy – a condition caused by hyperglycaemia where the nephrons of the kidney are damaged, impairing function. It is defined as a persistent and clinically detectable level of protein in the urine in association with an elevated blood pressure and reduced kidney function.

Niacin – vitamin B3.

Nocturnal hypoglycaemia – a fall in BG levels when you are asleep.

Normal BG control – 5.0–8.3 mmol/L.

Obstructive sleep apnoea – a condition causing intermittent and continual cessation of breathing during sleep, leading to reduced oxygen levels in the blood.

Oedema – fluid that gathers in the lower legs.

Over-active thyroid gland – where the thyroid gland at the front of the neck produces too much thyroid hormone that controls metabolism and growth.

Orlistat – Xenical – a medication that stops around one-third of the fat eaten from being digested.

Orthotist – a specially trained person at a hospital who makes made-to-measure shoes.

Osteoarthritis – degeneration of the joint cartilage and underlying bone causing pain and stiffness.

Osteopenia – refers to a reduction in bone mass.

Paediatric – relating to children.

PALS – Patient and Liaison Service.

Pancreas – a large organ lying behind the stomach that secretes digestive enzymes. Embedded within the pancreas are the *Islets of Langerhans*, which produce insulin.

Pantothenic acid – vitamin B5.

PCV – Passenger Carrying Vehicle.

Peripheral neuropathy – a chronic complication of diabetes occurring in two forms: diffuse neuropathy, appearing as disorders of sensation in the extremities of the body; and distal polyneuropathy, affecting many nerves of the hands and feet.

Peripheral vascular disease – a circulation disorder that causes blood vessels to become blocked. This can happen in arteries and veins.

Potassium – a mineral that's vital for the healthy function of body cells, tissues and organs and helps control water balance and blood acidity level in the body. It is found in bananas, avocados, spinach, lentils and all fruit and vegetables.

Poor BG control – 9.0 mmol/L and above.

Pre-diabetes (also known as insulin resistance) – defined as blood glucose concentrations higher than normal, but lower than established limits for diabetes itself.

Prednisone – anti-inflammatory medication.

Primary care – the healthcare you receive from your GP.

Prolactin – a hormone released from the anterior pituitary gland that stimulates milk production after childbirth.

Protein – any of a large group of compounds essential for growth as they are the building blocks of the body.

Psoriasis – an auto-immune condition that affects the skin and joints, causing red, flaky, crusty patches covered with silvery scales appearing on the elbows, knees, scalp and lower back, and joint degeneration. These skin patches can become itchy and sore.

Psychosis – a severe mental disorder where thoughts and emotions are impaired.

Pyridoxine – vitamin B6.

Rapid-acting insulin – a group of insulins for the treatment of Type 1 diabetes including Humalog, Novolog and Apidra, taken before meals to cover the associated BG rise. This is used with long-acting insulin and it takes 10–30 minutes to reach the bloodstream, where it works for three to five hours.

Reactive hypoglycaemia – low BG levels caused by the pancreas producing too much insulin in reaction, for example, to eating a meal. This does not happen in people with Type 1 diabetes.

RDA – Recommended Daily Allowance of vitamins and minerals.

Reduced absorption surgery – where the stomach is re-shaped by having around 80 per cent of it removed.

Restrictive surgery – as with reduced absorption surgery to the stomach, restrictive surgery works by physically making the size of the stomach much smaller to slow down digestion to give a feeling of fullness for longer with less food.

Retinopathy – a chronic complication of diabetes describing a number of symptoms including abnormal dilation of the blood vessels of the eyes, and bleeds in the retina at the back of the eyes. In advanced cases, the retina becomes heavily scarred and may lead to blindness.

Retinal photography – screening the eyes for diabetic retinopathy involves regular examinations to detect any diabetic changes that could affect sight. These changes are known as *sight-threatening diabetic retinopathy*. Retinal photography will decide whether you need follow-up treatment from the hospital eye clinic for diabetic retinopathy. If you have no diabetic changes, or if your existing retinopathy is stable, you will be asked to come back for screening a year later.

Retinol – the animal form of vitamin A.

Riboflavin – vitamin B2.

Roaccutane – a synthetic vitamin A supplement, also called *Isotretinoin*, that has been associated with birth defects when taken in large dosages of 25,000–500,000 international units per day.

Rosiglitazone – a medication used to lower BG levels in Type 2 diabetes.

Sedentary lifestyle – taking little or no exercise.

Self-efficacy – the self-confidence to do things, like using a BG testing machine, or drawing up and injecting insulin, and building on this to know you can tackle similar challenges.

Sensory nerve damage – diabetic changes to the sensory nerves affecting the ability to feel vibrations, temperature changes and gentle touches to the skin.

Serotonin – a hormone that gives us a sense of wellbeing.

Short-acting insulin – a group of insulins used to treat Type 1 diabetes including Regular (R) insulin taken 30 minutes before a meal to cover the rise in BG. This is used with long-acting insulin and takes 30 minutes to 1 hour to reach the blood stream, where it works for twelve hours.

Shoulder adhesive capsulitis – a chronic complication of diabetes describing a condition causing extreme pain and limited movement because the joint capsule has thickened and connective tissue becomes attached to the head of the humerus.

Statins – medication prescribed to lower cholesterol levels.

Stress response – something that makes the palms sweat; causes heart palpitations; headache and/or diarrhoea; tightness in the throat; tension; agitation; nausea; irritation; or short-temper. Emotionally this causes anxiety; unease; worry; panic; anger; or frustration.

Sugar – a simple carbohydrate that breaks down into glucose in the body.

Sulphonylureas – a group of medications used to reduce BG levels in people with Type 2 diabetes including Glimepiride – Amaryl; Glyburide – Diabetea, Micronase; Glipizide – Glucotrol, Glucotrol XL; Micronized Glyburide – Glynase.

Testosterone – the male sex hormone that, in men, stimulates the production of sperm and the development and maintenance of the appearance of male characteristics.

Thiamine – vitamin B1.

Thiazide – diuretic 'water' tablets that make you urinate more, which can increase BG levels.

Thiazollidines – a group of BG-lowering medications used to treat Type 2 diabetes including Pioglitazone (TZD) and Pioglitazone (Actos).

Thrush – common yeast infection of the vagina that affects most women, especially with diabetes, owing to raised BG levels. It occurs in warm, moist parts of the body and can also affect the throat – and some men, especially with diabetes.

Transient ischaemia – a partial restriction in blood supply to the brain.

Type 1 diabetes – a condition caused by auto-immune attack on the insulin-producing cells of the pancreas resulting in little or no insulin being available to lower BG levels.

Type 2 diabetes – a condition arising from metabolic syndrome where too much insulin is produced that the body can't use to reduce BG levels.

Under-active thyroid gland – a reduction in the amount of thyroid hormone produced by the thyroid gland in the neck.

Unexplained hypoglycaemia – low BG levels that happen for no reason and can't be linked, for example, to exercise, alcohol, drugs, aspirin or reactive hypoglycaemia.

Visceral fat – fat around the large internal organs of the abdomen.

Vitiligo – a condition where the pigmentation of the skin is lost in Type 1 diabetes as part of the body's auto-immune response to the condition.

Xanthelasma – a skin condition associated with diabetes where small yellow areas (plaques) appear on the eyelids and other areas of skin, which may be an indication of high blood fat (triglyceride) levels.

Bibliography

INTRODUCTION

Diabetes UK (2019), 'Us, diabetes and a lot of facts and stats'
https://www.diabetes.org.uk/resources-s3/2019-02/1362B_Facts%20
and%20stats%20Update%20Jan%202019_LOW%20RES_EXTERNAL.
pdf

Diabetes UK (2008), *Early Identification of Type 2 Diabetes and the new Vascular Risk Assessment and Management Programme*. Position Statement Update. (London: Diabetes UK).

Morgan, M. (2004), 'The evolution of the nutritional management of diabetes', *Proceedings of the Nutrition Society* 63, pp.615–20.

Willis, T. (1678), *Pharmaceutice Rationalis or an Excitation of the Operations of Medicines in Human Bodies* (London: Dring, Harper and Leigh).

Wilson, V. L. (2013), 'Type 2 diabetes in children and adolescents: a growing epidemic', *Nursing Children and Young People* 25(2), pp.14–17.

LIVING WITH DIABETES

American Diabetes Association (2003), 'Physical activity/exercise and diabetes mellitus', *Diabetes Care* 26(1), S73–S77.

BMI calculator: check your body mass index, patient.info/doctor/bmi-calculator.

Bree, A. J., Puente, E. C., Dorit, D-L., et al. (2009), 'Diabetes increases brain damage caused by severe hypoglycaemia', *American Journal of Physiology, Endocrinology and Metabolism* 297, E194–E201.

Colberg, S., Sigal, R., Ferhall, B., et al. (2010), 'Exercise and Type 2 diabetes', *Diabetes Care* 33(12), pp.2692–6.

Diabetes diagnosis (2017), www.diabetes.co.uk/Diabetes.diagnosis.html

'Diabetes and heredity: Genetic risk and other factors' (2017), www.medical-newstoday.com/articles/317468

Gabriel, I., Xiao, H.M., Xiao, M.Y., et al. (2002), 'Removal of visceral fat prevents insulin resistance and glucose intolerance of ageing', *Diabetes* 51(10), pp.2951–8.

Gray, N., Picone, G., Sloan, F., et al. (2015), 'The relationship between BMI and onset of diabetes mellitus and its complications', *Journal of Southern Medicine* 108(1), pp.29–36.

Hikino, H. (1991), 'Traditional remedies and modern assessment; The case of ginseng'. In Wijeskera, R. O. B. (ed.), *The Medical Plant Industry* (Boca Ration, Florida: CRC Press), pp.149–66.

Holford, P. (1992), *Optimum Nutrition: How to Get the Very Best Out of Yourself* (London: ION Press).

Weyer, C., et al. (2001), 'Hypoadioponectinemia in obesity and Type 2 diabetes: Close association with insulin resistance and hyperinsulinaemia', *The Journal of Clinical Endocrinology and Metabolism* 86(5), pp.1930–5.

Marks, V., & Richmond, C. (2007), *Insulin Murders: True Life Cases* (London: Royal Society of Medicine Press Limited).

'What medicines can make your blood sugar spike?' (2017) https://www.webmd.com/diabetes/medicines-blood-sugar-spike

'Steps to take if your oral diabetes medication stops working' www.healthline.com/health/type-2-diabetes/oral-medication-stops-working

'The DVLA and diabetes – find out what you need to know' https://www.diabetes.org.uk/Guide-to-diabetes/Life-with-diabetes/Driving?gclid=EAIaIQobChMI8N6clLmp4QIVWfhRCh3cOgPoEAAYAS AAEgLmKfD_BwE

Wellen, K. E., & Hotamisligil, G. S. (2005), 'Inflammation, stress and diabetes', *The Journal of Clinical Investigation* 115(5), pp.1111–19.

Wilson, V. L. (2012), 'Evaluation of the care received by older people with diabetes', *Nursing Older People* 24(4), pp.33–7.

Wilson, V. L. (2006), 'Diabetes and older people: Issues of diagnosis and care', *Journal of Diabetes Nursing* 10(5), pp.182–5.

A ROLLERCOASTER OF EMOTIONS

Biddle, S. J., Fox, K. R., & Boutcher, S. H. (eds.) (2000), *Physical Activity and Psychological Well-Being.* (New York: Routledge).

Bishop, G. D., Smelser, N. J., & Baltes, P. B. (2001), *Emotions and Health* (Oxford: Pergamon).

Clark, M. (2004a), *Understanding Diabetes.* (West Sussex, England: John Wiley & Sons Ltd).

Bulut, A., & Bulut., A. (2016), 'Evaluation of anxiety condition among type 1 and type 2 diabetic patients', *Neuropsychiatric Disease Treatment* 12, pp.2573–9.

Clark, M. (2004b), 'Identification and treatment of depression in people with diabetes', *Diabetes and Primary Care* 5(3), pp.124–7.

Fisher, L., Mullan, J. T., Arean, P., et al. (2010), 'Diabetes distress but not clinical depression or depressive symptoms is associated with glycemic control in both cross-sectional and longitudinal analyses', *Diabetes Care* 33, pp.23–8.

Gask, L., Macdonald, W., & Bower, P. (2011), 'What is the relationship between diabetes and depression? A qualitative meta-synthesis of patient experience of co-morbidity', *Chronic Illness* 7, pp.239–52.

Izard, C. E. (2007), 'Basic emotions, natural kinds, emotion schemas, and a new paradigm', *Perspectives on Psychological Science* 2, pp.260–80.

Brehm, J. & Brummet, B. (1998), 'The emotional control of behavior'. In Kofta, M., Weary, G., & Sedek G. (eds.), *Personal Control in Action* (Springer), pp.133–54.

Piette, J. D., Richardson, C., & Valenstein, M. (2004), 'Addressing the needs of patients with multiple chronic illness: the case of diabetes and depression', *The American Journal of Managed Care* 10(2), pp.152–64.

Rush, W. A., Whitebird, R. R., Rush, M. R., et al. (2008), 'Depression in patients with diabetes: Does it impact clinical goals?', *Journal of the American Board of Family Medicine* 21(5), pp.392–7.

Wax, R. (2013), *Sane New World: Taming the Mind* (Croydon: Hodder & Stoughton).

HOW WILL DIABETES AFFECT ME?

Adams, O. P. (2013), 'The impact of brief high-intensity exercise on blood glucose levels', *Diabetes, Metabolic Syndrome, and Obesity* 6, pp.113–22.

'Calories burned' (2018)
www.healthstatus.com/calculate/cbc

'Exercise' (2018)
www.nhs.uk/live-well/exercise/

'Facts on alternative blood sugar testing sites' (2018)
https://www.verywellhealth.com/alternate-blood-sugar-testing-sites-3289624

Gill, D. L., Hammons, C. C., Reifsteck, E. J., et al. (2013), 'Physical activity and quality of life', *Journal of Preventative Medicine and Public Health* 46 (Supplement 1), S28–S34.

Hammadi, S. H., Al-Ghamdi, S. S., Yassian, A. I., et al. (2012), 'Aspirin and blood glucose and insulin resistance', *Open Journal of Endocrine and Metabolic Diseases* 2, pp.16–26.

HbA1c units converter (2018)
http://www.wales.nhs.uk/sitesplus/documents/866/HbA1c%20converter.pdf

Steiner, J. L., Crowell, K. T., & Lang, C. H. (2015), 'Impact of alcohol on gly-caemia control and insulin action', *Biomolecules* 5(4), pp.2223–46.

'Symptoms of low blood sugar' (2018)
https://www.nhs.uk/conditions/low-blood-sugar-hypoglycaemia/

Wilson, V. L. (2012a), 'Diagnosis and treatment of diabetic ketoacidosis', *Emergency Nursing* 20(7), pp.14–18.

Wilson, V. L. (2012b), 'Reflections on reducing insulin to lose weight', *Nursing Times* 108(43), pp.21–5.

Wilson, V. L. (2011), 'Non-diabetic hypoglycaemia: causes and pathophysiol-ogy', *Nursing Standard* 25(46), pp.35–40.

Wilson, V. L. (2010), 'Type 1 diabetes self-management: a patient's experience of CGMS' (Letter to the Editor), *European Diabetes Nursing* 7(1), p.15.

LIFESTYLE CHANGE

'Diabetes education: knowing more about your condition'
https://www.diabetes.org.uk/guide-to-diabetes/managing-your-diabetes/education

Diabetes UK (2011), 'Carbohydrate reference list'
https://www.diabetes.org.uk/resources-s3/2017-11/carb-reference-list-0511.pdf

'Essential guide to fats' (2018) https://www.bhf.org.uk/informationsupport/support/healthy-living/healthy-eating/fats-explained

'Glycaemic index and diabetes' (2016)
https://beyondtype1.org/glycemic-index-diet-diabetes/?gclid=EAIaIQobChMIo8H2-L-p4QIV5BbTCh2P7AblEAAYAiAAEgKU8vD_BwE

Harrar, S. (2011), 'Taking diabetes drugs with nutritional supplements', *Today's Dietician* 13(11), p.32.

Rubin, A. L., & Jarvis, S. (2011), *Diabetes for Dummies* (London: John Wiley & Sons Ltd).

'Understanding food labels' (2018)
https://www.diabetes.org.uk/guide-to-diabetes/enjoy-food/food-shopping-for-diabetes/understanding-food-labels

'What does 100 calories look like?' (2018)
https://www.nhs.uk/live-well/eat-well/what-does-100-calories-look-like/

'Why 5 a Day?' (2017)
https://www.nhs.uk/live-well/eat-well/why-5-a-day/

GETTING BACK CONTROL – MANAGING DIABETES AND SELF-MEDICATION

'Diabetes medication side effects' (2019)
www.diabetes.co.uk/features/diabetes-medication-side-effects.html

'Inhaled insulin: Can I take insulin without a needle?' (2017)
https://www.webmd.com/diabetes/inhaled-insulin

'Insulin injection sites: Where and how to inject insulin' (2017)
www.healthline.com/health/diabetes/insulin-injection

'List of common diabetes medications' (2018)
www.healthline.com/health/diabetes/medications-list

National Institute for Health and Care Excellence (2019), 'Insulin: Treatment summary'
bnf.nice.org.uk/treatment-summary/insulin-2.html

National Institute for Health and Care Excellence (2008), 'Continuous sub-cutaneous insulin infusion for the treatment of diabetes mellitus'.
www.nice.org.uk/guidance/ta151

Wilson, V. L. (2007), 'Perceived support needs for intensive diabetes self-management', *Journal of Diabetes Nursing* 11(1), pp.8–13.

Wilson, V. L. (2005), 'Complications of diabetes: human and healthcare costs', *Journal of Diabetes Nursing* 9(4), pp.133–6.

KNOW YOUR ENEMY!

'Autoimmune diseases' (2018)
https://medlineplus.gov/autoimmunediseases.html

'How to look after your feet' (2017)
https://www.diabetes.org.uk/guide-to-diabetes/complications/feet/taking-care-of-your-feet

Krzewska, A., & Ben-Skowronek, I. (2016), 'Effect of associated auto-immune diseases on Type 1 diabetes mellitus in children and adolescents', *Biomedical Research.*
https://www.ncbi.nlm.nih.gov/pubmed/27525273

'Medications that can raise blood sugar (glucose) levels' (2017)
https://www.webmd.com/diabetes/medicines-blood-sugar-spike

'National screening programme for diabetic retinopathy' (2014)
www.nscretinopathy.org.uk

Ward, S. A. (2005), 'Diabetes, exercise, and foot care: minimizing risks in patients who have neuropathy'.
www.ncbi.nlm.nih.gov/pubmed/20086374

Wilson, V. L. (2012a), 'Myocardial infarction symptoms and appropriate action: awareness of people with diabetes', *British Journal of Cardiac Nursing* 7(6), pp.287–92.

Wilson, V. L. (2012b), 'Cognitive impairment in patients with diabetes', *Nursing Standard* 27, pp.15–17.

Wilson, V. L. (2006a), 'Preventing retinopathy with regular screening and effective treatment', *British Journal of Primary Care Nursing* 3(1), pp.21–3.

Wilson, V. L. (2006b), 'The experience of a person living with peripheral neuropathy,' *Journal of Diabetes Nursing* 10(7), pp.256–8.

DIABETES TRAINING COURSES

'How do I access a DAFNE course?' Find your nearest DAFNE centre: http://www.dafne.uk.com/all-courses.html

DESMOND – Diabetes Education and Self-Management for Ongoing and Newly Diagnosed
www.diabetes.co.uk/education/desmond.html

Your nearest DESMOND centre
www.desmond-project.org.uk/people-with-diabetes/

'How am I feeling?' In *Resources for You* (2010)
www.desmond-project.org.uk

'Burn 100 calories'
https://www.sparkpeople.com/resource/fitness_articles.asp?id=1777

REVERSING TYPE 2 DIABETES

Browne, J. L., Ventura, A., Mosley, K., et al. (2017), '"I call it the blame and shame disease": a qualitative study about perceptions of social stigma surrounding type 2 diabetes', *British Medical Journal* 3(11).
bmjopen.bmj.com/content/3/11/e003384

National Institute for Health and Care Excellence (NICE) (2014a), 'The management of Type 2 diabetes'.
www.nice.org.uk/guidance/cg87

National Institute for Health and Care Excellence (NICE) (2014c), 'Obesity identification assessment and management of overweight and obesity in children, young people and adults'.
www.nice.org.uk/guidance/cg189

Rubiano, F. (2006b), 'Bariatric surgery: effects on glucose homeostasis', *Current Opinion in Clinical Nutrition and Metabolic Care* 9, pp.497–507.

Weight loss surgery: Availability – NHS
https://www.nhs.uk/conditions/weight-loss-surgery/

Wilson, V. L. (2015), 'Reversing Type 2 diabetes with lifestyle change', *Nursing Times* 111(12), pp.17–19.

WHAT DIABETES CARE SHOULD I RECEIVE?

Annual diabetes checks (2017)
https://www.diabetes.org.uk/guide-to-diabetes/managing-your-diabetes/15-healthcare-essentials

Diabetes care and you (2017)
https://www.diabetes.org.uk/resources-s3/2017-11/diabetescareandyou_final_8010.pdf

Diabetes clinics (2017)
https://www.diabetes.org.uk/guide-to-diabetes/young-adults/diabetes-clinics

Diabetes inpatients and hospital care (2016)
https://www.diabetes.org.uk/professionals/resources/shared-practice/inpatient-and-hospital-care

Making a complaint about healthcare (2017)
https://www.nhs.uk/using-the-nhs/about-the-nhs/how-to-complain-to-the-nhs/

Meet your healthcare team (2017)
https://www.diabetes.org.uk/guide-to-diabetes/managing-your-diabetes/
interactions-with-healthcare-professionals

What care to expect (2016)
https://www.diabetes.org.uk/guide-to-diabetes/teens/me-and-my-diabetes/
healthcare/what-care-to-expect

YOUNG AND OLD

'Avoiding hypos' (2018)
https://www.diabetes.org.uk/guide-to-diabetes/kids/me-and-my-diabetes/
getting-my-glucose-right/hypos/avoiding-hypos

'Caring for someone with diabetes – Elderly, children, partner' (2017)
www.diabetes.co.uk/caring-for-someone-with-diabetes.html

'Checking blood glucose in newborn babies' (2016)
https://www.caringforkids.cps.ca/handouts/blood_glucose_in_newborn_
babies

Diabetes UK (2019), 'Us, diabetes, and a lot of facts and stats'
https://www.diabetes.org.uk/resources-s3/2019-02/1362B_Facts%20and%20
stats%20Update%20Jan%202019_LOW%20RES_EXTERNAL.pdf

'Meal plans and diabetes' (for Parents) (2017)
kidshealth.org/en/parents/meal-plans-diabetes.html

'What is the honeymoon period in Type 1 diabetes?' (2018)
www.healthline.com/health/diabetes/honeymoon-period-diabetes

Wilson, V. L. (2013), 'Type 2 diabetes in children and adolescents: a growing
epidemic,' *Nursing Children and Young People* 25(2), pp.14–17.

Wilson, V. L. (2012), 'Evaluation of the care received by older people with
diabetes,' *Nursing Older People* 24(4), pp.33–7.

Wilson, V. L. (2010), 'Students managing type 1 diabetes', *Paediatric Nursing* 22(10), pp.25–8.

Wilson, V. L. (2008), 'Experiences of parents of young people with diabetes using insulin pump therapy', *Paediatric Nursing* 20(2), pp.14–18.

Wilson, V. L., & Beskine, D. (2007), 'Children and young people with diabetes: managing at school', *Journal of Diabetes Nursing* 11(10), pp.392–8.

Wilson, V. L., & Beskine, D. (2007), 'Pump therapy in the management of children and young people with type 1 diabetes', *Journal of Diabetes Nursing* 11(9), pp.352–7.

Wilson, V. L. (2006), 'Diabetes and older people: Issues of diagnosis and care', *Journal of Diabetes Nursing* 10(5), pp.182–5.

World Health Organisation (2018), 'Ageing and health'
https://www.who.int/news-room/fact-sheets/detail/ageing-and-health

HELPFUL HINTS AND TIPS

Friends, family and diabetes
www.cdc.gov/features/diabetes-family-friends/index.html

'Ten ways to get others to help you'
Jarvis, S. & Rubin, A. (2003), *Diabetes for Dummies* (London: John Wiley & Sons Ltd).

Index